Daring Docs

Daring Docs

✦

High Drama in *Journal AMA* Papers and Other Investigative Reporting

Milton Golin

ASJA Press
New York Lincoln Shanghai

Daring Docs

High Drama in *Journal AMA* Papers and Other Investigative Reporting

ASJA Press
an imprint of iUniverse, Inc.

iUniverse books may be ordered through booksellers or by contacting:

iUniverse
2021 Pine Lake Road, Suite 100
Lincoln, NE 68512
www.iuniverse.com
1-800-Authors (1-800-288-4677)

Exclusive True Stories of Survival Without Heartbeat, Disaster MDs, Mars Rescue Plan, Life-Saving Serendipity, Teen Therapists, Foiled Assassination, Armed Mutiny

ISBN-13: 978-0-595-38194-4 (pbk)
ISBN-13: 978-0-595-82563-9 (ebk)
ISBN-10: 0-595-38194-4 (pbk)
ISBN-10: 0-595-82563-X (ebk)

Printed in the United States of America

"Get it right...If your mother says she loves you, check it out"

—Oft-quoted accuracy admonition to City News Bureau of Chicago reporters

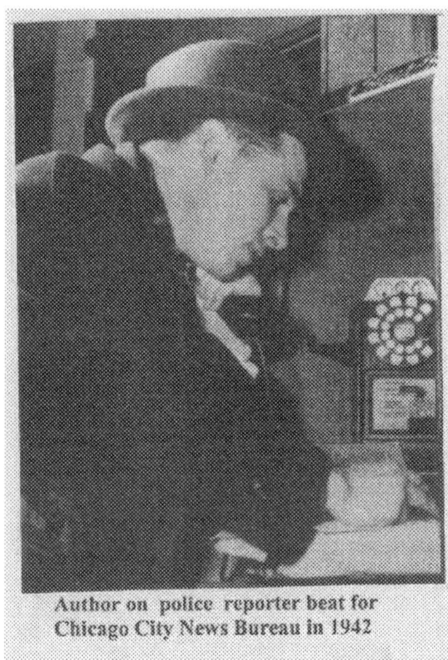
Author on police reporter beat for Chicago City News Bureau in 1942

* At midnight on December 31, 2005, after more than a century of continuous operation, City News Bureau finally closed its doors.

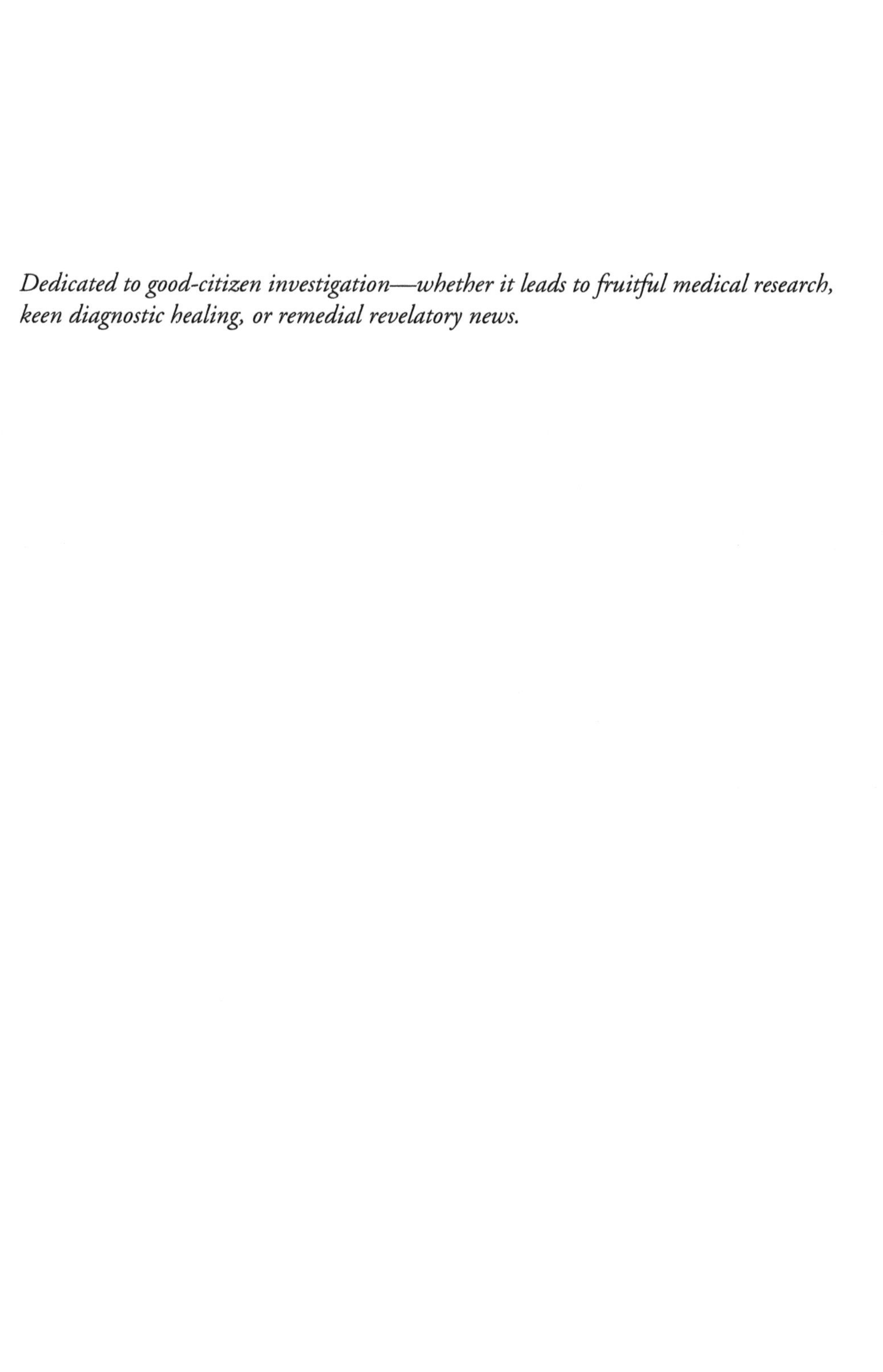

Dedicated to good-citizen investigation—whether it leads to fruitful medical research, keen diagnostic healing, or remedial revelatory news.

Contents

Introduction

Recalling the events of 9/11, what if someone on your airplane was going to kill you and everyone else on board?

What if an operating room patient cheats death after his heart apparently stops beating for an incredible two and a half hours?

What if heroism on a grand scale marks the activity of 40 doctors in a lethal hurricane?

What if two leading aerospace scientists theorize the rescue of a future astronaut whose space capsule crashes on the surface of Mars?

What if the missing immigrant who saved Theodore Roosevelt from assassination in 1912 turns up in a reporter's search for him 38 years later?

What if a Denver man arrested for dynamiting an airliner unnerves the warden by abruptly describing in a jailhouse interview how the FBI framed him?

What if you watch aghast as overloaded warplanes crash and burn?

Daring Docs is not about what-ifs, not fictional scenes. These and other true episodes, some of them reported in *The Journal of the American Medical Association* and elsewhere, are confronted, probed, noted, logged, taped, photographed, drawn, memorized, developed, and written by a wide-ranging investigative journalist.

Saga of the Disaster Doctors

The catastrophic hurricane Katrina that crippled most of New Orleans and surrounding areas on August 29, 2005 magnified a less-devastating but nevertheless horrible Louisiana hurricane 48 years earlier. Then, in similar bayou country, were similar victims on rooftops, similar vermin-ridden and swirling floodwaters, similar hero rescuers, and similar personal consternations A big difference: preparedness in the earlier storm.

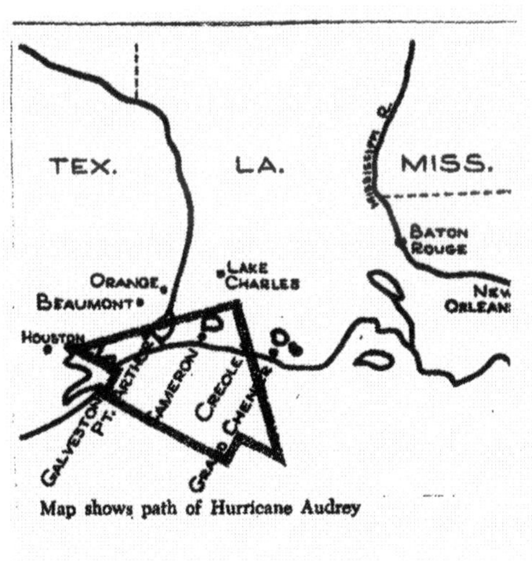

Map shows path of Hurricane Audrey

In broadcasting stations and newspaper offices on June 25, 1957, United Press Teletypes are clattering a weather advisory, then another and another. The wicked hurricane "Audrey" was then only a "tropical disturbance" setting a course toward landfall on the Gulf Coast of western Louisiana and eastern Texas.

But 40 physicians, fresh from a U.S. civil defense briefing session at their Calcasieu Parish Medical Society meeting in a Lake Charles, LA restaurant, do not know this yet. Hardly anybody does. It is past midnight and the bayou country is asleep.

Wednesday, June 26, dawns much as the day before. Morning papers and radio newscasts are informing communities at their breakfast table that a big storm is coming. Most folks, many of them French-speaking, are not alarmed; they have seen bad weather before. But some are worried. Cameron Parish Sheriff O. B. Carter, warning residents of Cameron, Creole, and Grand Chenier to evacuate, describes these towns as "nothing but hills in the swamp." Only a few of the coastal residents begin getting ready to leave the area.

In adjoining Texas, though, there is consternation. That state's middle name has been catastrophe: first in the nation in number of all disasters (some 250 in the past year, killing over 1,000 persons in the last decade alone), first in tornadoes, second in hurricanes, first in devastating floods.

And as the news reports come in, memories are still fresh—of the Dallas tornado of April 2, the Lampasas flood of May 12 (said to be the worst in recent Texas history), the Silverton tornado of May 16. Only 10 of the state's 254 counties can boast they have not been eligible for federal disaster aid since 1950.

Late that night on June 26 in Port Arthur, Texas, a 39-year-old surgeon, Dr. Robert S. Browne, reads in his newspaper that the storm might bring a 5-to-9-foot tidal wave by noon next day. He is ready to help. Across the river in Cameron, LA, 33-year-old Dr. Cecil W. Clark, living the life of a typical country doctor on native soil, reviews his day's work.

He had waved goodbye to his three children at home four miles east of Cameron (two other youngsters were at his mother's home outside the area), and that day he had been first to set eyes on three other children, babies he delivered in his 12-bed clinic hospital. There in Cameron, Dr. Clark comforts the new mothers and another patient, a man recovering from an injured knee.

Fifteen miles away in Creole, LA, 30-year-old Dr. Stephen E. Carter is thinking of his family. And 36-year-old Dr. George W. Dix, peering at the sky, is wondering how a bachelor like himself might find a planned medical practice in Africa under these conditions. A lover of remote, semitropical nature, he picked Creole because it seemed to have some of Africa's primitiveness. In the Lake Charles Memorial Hospital, Administrator Joseph W. Hinsley, who is also the civil defense coordinator, stays up for the latest newscast. It says the storm is moving at seven miles an hour toward Galveston and is due to hit the coastal region late the next day, June 27. It is 1 a.m. and the storm, turning into a whip, is due to hit Lake Charles in full force at noon, eight hours ahead of schedule.

By 3 a.m. more than 20 physicians and nurses who were supposed to assemble after dawn are in the hospital lobby, ready for action. Not many are sleepy-eyed as they take stock of cots and stretchers, order extra supplies of food and oxygen, distribute linens and medical supplies, and arrange for filling several thousand milk cartons with water.

Large windows are braced and taped, roof hatches battened down, the hospital's electric generator is hooked up. Elective [optional] surgery is cancelled, and convalescents able to do so are urged to return home.

Dawn manages to outrace the wind. At Memorial Hospital in Lake Charles, 12 babies are born in the next 24 hours, two on stretcher carts during the height of the hurricane. In Cameron, meanwhile, Dr. Clark's wife huddles with her three children as the hurricane whirls in at 110 miles an hour. Her husband had left their home earlier, after a 2 a.m. phone report of water reaching his hospital and patients.

By the time he gets there, the clinic is gone; it has been picked up and deposited in a marsh a mile and a half away. The office of Cameron Parish's only other physician, Stephen E. Carter, also is destroyed in the waters sweeping over Creole.

It is now approaching noon in relatively plush Lake Charles. Hurricane Audrey announces her arrival by smashing a braced 6-by-12-ft. Memorial Hospital window. Glass spatters over administrator Hensley and onto a half-dozen large pans of food set on a steam table for lunch. So the dining room is evacuated, the menu is changed to cold cuts, and Hinsley's head is bandaged.

Just before dawn, a 200-bed portable civil defense hospital unit unloads onto floating "ducks" for the trek southward. Along goes Hensley, his assistant, a dozen physicians, and 16 nurses. They pass through the most devastated country any of them had ever seen.

Dead cattle float past them, other animals stand marooned on small patches of roadway. Fallen electrical wires and debris block the caravan's path from time to time. Low-hanging power cables injure a male nurse and a photographer when they fail to duck in time. In an hour the party stops at Gibbstown to give first aid. They continue to Creole, or what is left of it.

There is no place to assemble the hospital unit except in the road, on a site practically surrounded by water. So that's where they organize medical headquarters. It is done in 30 minutes. (Without previous rehearsals and color-scheming of parts, it would have taken about five hours to set up.) With a base established, the watery caravan splits up.

One contingent of "ducks" heads for Cameron and another in the opposite direction for Grand Chenier. Physicians owning their own boats shuttle supplies to both towns and bring back refugees to Creole and Lake Charles. Many of the injured are treated and tagged before evacuation.

It is clear now there must have been panic among thousands of residents in the three communities strung parallel to the coast, since the tidal wave had washed directly across the only good road connecting the three towns. There is no dry escape to the north.

Another dawn breaks at Lake Charles, illuminating the Coast Guard ship Bluebonnet as it arrives with the first survivors—41 men, women, and some children whose faces still wear the shock of seeing whole families wiped out, communities smashed, victims screaming as they hang from rooftops, barbed wire fences, and tree limbs.

At first, some of the accounts are incredible to doctors and nurses at a designated casualty sorting center in the McNeese State College gymnasium in St. Charles. But as the refugees stumble in, the grim reality begins to take hold.

Noon approaches. Medical field headquarters at Creole is a busy scene as survivors are treated for shock, fractures, and other injuries. Suddenly the chatter on a civil defense radio receiver is interrupted by a loud voice reporting to a headquarters somewhere: "We have called for help from doctors in Texas. There are no Louisiana doctors at distress areas in Cameron parish."

Hinsley boils inside, wishing he could set the record straight, but his radio transmitter isn't working. One doctor quips, "What does that guy think we're doing here, cracking pecans?"

Just about this time, the telephone rings in Dr. Robert Browne's office in Port Arthur, Texas. It is the local radio station. They, too, have heard the erroneous report that no Louisiana doctors are on duty along the coast and that Texas physicians are needed.

Would Dr. Browne board a shrimp trawler to bring supplies to Cameron? He would. Moments later an announcer broadcasts the news and it is heard in Port Arthur by another surgeon, 37-year-old Thomas B. "Tony" Sappington Jr.

Several hours later, when news of the "emergency" reaches Beaumont, 38-year-old internist Darwin D. Moore and an assistant physician in that city's tuberculosis hospital, Dr. M. T. Danak, a native of India, climb into a Sun Oil Company plane for the trip to Cameron. Obstetrician Lewis M. Williams, 35, drives there from his Beaumont office.

In Louisiana, meanwhile, every physician in Calcasieu and Cameron parishes is on disaster duty. They include the three Cameron parish doctors who have lost their homes and clinic buildings under swirling water. Not until Friday afternoon does Dr. Clark hear that his wife and three children are believed drowned.

(Later, Mrs. Clark is found safe, but the children are dead—the youngest, three-and-a-half-year-old Jack, having been torn from her arms by a huge wave;

two other children survive in their grandmother's home.) Though stricken, Dr. Clark spends the next few days treating flood victims and directing emergency medical work at the courthouse refuge.

After all, isn't he Cameron's only resident physician? He explains later: "I figured my place was with those who were hurt. I would have to put my family temporarily in the background." A deputy sheriff says, "The doctor was tired and had a sad look on his face. He was broken-hearted and the people really appreciated what he has done."

It takes five hours for the shrimp boat carrying Drs. Browne and Sappington to tie up at the Cameron jetties as Hurricane Audrey ebbs sullenly back to sea. Dr. Browne recalls: "There were just us four doctors at first in the courthouse—Tony Sappington, myself, internist John K. Griffith Jr. from Lake Charles, and Dr. White from Alexandria, who had been visiting in Lake Charles and came along to help.

"We worked by lanterns, flashlights, candles. There were tetanus and typhoid shots to give, fractures to reduce, lives to save. One fellow dared me to inoculate him. I said it was up to him, that he was risking his life. He still refused.

"We even had a gunshot case. Tony Sappington treated an 18-year-old youth who had been wounded by a rifle bullet during an argument over whether he with a shotgun or another teenager with a rifle was better armed as a deputy sheriff to prevent looting in Cameron. Both lost their deputy status and had to be evacuated. We had some snakebite cases, too."

Snakes are a terrifying hazard. The bayous are full of ground rattlers and water moccasins. They slither onto debris, snapping at human refugees beside them. Mrs. Stephen Broussard loses three children to the tidal wave, and a fourth dies when a snake strikes as she is holding the child in the water.

Dr. Danak, just in from Beaumont, has cause to dwell on the scene as a reminder of his native India, where countrymen on rooftops during monsoon floods would often choose a watery suicide than submit to the nerve-killing attacks of also-marooned kraits. Even more terrifying, at least in appearance, are the nutria muskrats, some weighing up to 25 pounds. They bare long curved teeth when cornered. Several refugees bitten by these vicious rodents are treated at the Cameron treatment center.

Fifteen miles from the courthouse there, in the water-flanked open air portable hospital, snakebite cases come as no surprise.They had been expected in the civil defense plan. Physicians left Lake Charles with 75 snakebite kits, including 36 borrowed hastily from local Boy Scouts.

There seems to be no end to the misery, stink, and shock in Cameron. Bodies fill up the ice house. Dr. Browne of Beaumont, a former Texas National Guardsman, is familiar with disaster. As a boy in St. Louis, he witnessed the great Midwest tornado that killed over 400 persons in 1925; he had rushed gas masks and performed surgery for victims of the Texas City natural disaster in 1947 and two years ago helped organize medical help for flood victims in Orange TX.

On Saturday, Dr. Clark is flown by helicopter to Lake Charles for a reunion with his surviving wife and children. Although relief for the doctors from Texas and from Cameron and Calcasieu parishes is coming in from other localities, many of them stay on serving until Sunday evening—more than three days and three nights without regular sleep.

By then, the curtain of shock has lifted in many victims but the horrendous memories never can be erased. At the treatment centers people ask, "Have you any water?" Before the doctor can answer, they add: "I don't want any if someone needs it more than I do."

Now the bodies are decomposing quickly in the heat and humidity, and there are not enough disaster pouches in which to enclose them before heavy machinery can dig huge graves for mass burial. So there is a rush call for garment bags, mattress covers, even quickly sewn bed sheets.

Sunday, June 30, is the first day of assessment, although medical teams continue to give mass inoculations against typhoid and tetanus. Hurricane Audrey's toll is at least 518 dead in Louisiana with perhaps many more among entire transient workers' families who were washed out to sea, unidentified and unsought; nine dead in Texas; more than 1,000 injured, and many thousands made homeless in property damage totaling $48 million.

On July 12, when a make-believe enemy was supposed to have hit the center of Lake Charles with one atom bomb and an outlying Air Force base with another, Cameron parish civil defense director Larry W. Stephenson announces to doctors who had been alerted in June: "We are not expected to participate in the national civil defense exercise."

They have had it.

How Deadly the Thought

Although a hurricane in Louisiana wields death and destruction in a hard-hit part of the country, neurosis exerts a kind of human damage that is more widespread. It's like a sneeze resounding in a crowded elevator. A dozen people are in danger of catching a cold.

A teacher is reprimanded by a superior who had been in a nasty frame of mind after a tiff with his wife at breakfast. How "catching" is that mood? To what extent will the teacher, in turn, infect her pupils with resentment?

A series of magazine sketches portrays a frustrated boss yelling at a worker for supposed laxity. On returning home, the employee is shown castigating his wife for no apparent reason. She then scolds their young son for apparent misbehavior. Finally, we see the boy kicking the family cat.[1]

For many years, sociologists, philosophers, physicians, and clergymen have been trying to convey the point that an individual's attitude—whether it centers around a single thought or a complex of ideas—can be contagious. But how could the thesis be proved scientifically? How might the unique "airborne" spread of good or bad mental health be weighed in its elements, analyzed, and eventually controlled for the benefit mankind?

For the first time, as noted in *Charm* magazine,[2] speakers at a symposium described studies of the communicability of mental and emotional illness. Taking part were educators, physicians, sociologists, and anthropologists, led by the Joint Commission on Mental Illness and Health.

Participants in government agencies, educational institutions, and private medical practice devoted eight hours exploring the transmission and reception of such disorders. Later, the American Medical Association president had this to say: "We face in essence a heretofore unrecognized epidemic of mental and emotional illness throughout our country and the world. We need to understand what the susceptibility and resistance of our population is to these."

Dr. Jonas Salk told the same conference that when enough is known about the disorders, measures might be taken to immunize the healthy. "There is no reason to believe," he said, "that cells of the nervous system will not respond in the same way as cells that create immunity to polio. An individual is determined not by genes alone, but also by a number of events that occur after birth."

Where do these events occur? At home and in school, at work, and in social and recreational settings. They happen anywhere and everywhere that ideas and attitudes, both valid and twisted, impinge and reimpinge on human brains like ping pong balls on so many sounding boards. Here are some cases cited in the medical literature:

A Chicago businessman, preparing to file his income tax report, remarks facetiously, "Well, I may be able to beat the government out of some money." His young son, unable to discriminate between sarcasm and strict fact, places the remark in the recesses of his mind as license to do wrong elsewhere. In the same way, evidence indicates that injudicious adult comment about racial groups can be stored up for next-generation prejudice.

A well-known actress plays the role of a schizophrenic in a Hollywood movie, and months later is in a mental hospital still trying to stop playing the role. Commenting on this case of "autocommunicability"—catching an illness from oneself—a leading psychiatrist who more or less limits his practice to the emotional problems of film stars, says bluntly, "Three quarters of the Hollywood acting population is either insane, just getting over being insane, or about to go insane…They are highly paid for their fantasies and daydreams and often for their craziness. Let them get too well-adjusted, and there's no telling what might happen to their jobs."

Ten workers from the same department of an electronics firm show up at the dispensary in a short period of time—complaining of backaches, headaches, and other physical discomfort. "No cause you can pin down," the company physician reports. But a check reveals that their supervisor, disturbed over a family matter, had suddenly become strict and overbearing, and brief psycho-therapy was begun. Soon the supervisor is back in balance and the workers are all right, too.[2]

Those cases illuminate some of the seeds of communicability. They may be planted by person-to-person contact, be fertilized in the family to grow throughout the community, or be blown and sown from nation to nation. Contact might simply communicate a fleeting idea or involve the transference of broad patterns of thinking.

Under certain conditions, such contagion in its most harmful form could apply even to a psychosis. *Folie á deux* is one example of induced insanity that has been recognized by doctors for more than a century. Two French clinicians described it in 1877 as a "mental disorder in which symptoms, particularly paranoid delusion, from which one of two persons is suffering, are communicated to and accepted by the other."

An example of nonpsychotic communicability is the famous dancing mania, a behavioral disorder of the fourteenth century which caused thousands of people to dance uncontrollably in the streets of Europe. Sociologists also cite the goldfish-swallowing craze of the 1930's, the panty raids that spread from campus to campus, and other fads that bespeak a human readiness to follow the crowd.

Even the concept of "psychopathic nations," communicating a kind of derangement among themselves, has been noted in medicine. Dr. Jerome D. Frank, an associate professor of psychiatry at Johns Hopkins University, suggested during the Cold War that the United States and Russia "bred" dislike (as do paranoid patients) when the two governments become mutually suspicious and force each other to behave in a manner that confirms and heightens the others' fears.

Famed psychiatrist Dr. Will Menninger once pointed out it is ridiculous to believe that the carrier of a disease must necessarily be a physical, chemical, or biological thing. "An agent of disease," he says, "can be a bullet or it can be an idea. It can be persecution. It can be any number of things. Our problem may be due to a mixing of our value systems.

"We seem to be more effective in communicating our material goals than our spiritual goals. When I say a leader must understand people, I mean the kind of leader who has some understanding of personalities, their structure and function, how they work, and who knows of the unreasonableness in all of us, and hostilities we all have. We need a program to fight bigotry, hate, panic, smugness—contagious diseases of the mind that have shattered more societies than all the viruses known to civilization."

Going a step farther was Dr. Paul M. Kersten of Fort Dodge, Iowa. He told the conference on communicability that there is a "very direct correlation between the general level of emotional maturity in individual members of a given culture, and its decline." Of course, to assume that a mentally healthy person will, by mere association, automatically "catch" someone else's emotional illness is as absurd as to believe that tuberculosis is universally contagious. It is not. In fact, there is strong evidence that contact with the mentally ill can be therapeutic. Dr. Karl Menninger described the phenomenon:

"Many of our citizens (of Topeka, Kansas) have discovered that it is not only the sick who are benefited when a town gets interested in psychiatric illness. There is something about working with sick minds that makes ordinary people sensitive to suffering, more tolerant, more human—even to each other. They discover that love cures people, the ones who receive love and the ones who give it."

How, then, can people build a pattern of resistance that will make them stronger, instead of weaker, in the presence of mental or emotional disorder? One guidepost for them might well be the ability of an individual to discriminate between fact and fiction, between truths and half-truths. There is some solid evidence that, like an infectious smile, mental health can be catching. A child who is taught not to steal develops a feeling—not just an understanding—that creates an iron-clad prejudice against stealing.

A surgeon told the communicability conference about his experience: "I go to a hospital and am met by a cheerful doorman. Then I find a mentally healthy man at the head of the hospital. The whole place reflects his personality."

Another instance of mental "contagion" turned to positive good has been described by the Baltimore psychiatrist Dr. Leo Bartemeier. He told a group of insurance company employees who had worked morosely in adjoining cubby holes for years, without knowing or speaking to one another. One day they were assembled, introduced to one another, and encouraged to chat.

"These people developed a camaraderie, a sense of identification with the company, and with their fellow workers," said Dr. Bartemeier. "Each was enabled to see the other as a human being with desires and frustrations—not just a hand or a body."

The measure of that kind of mental health does not lie in inverse proportion to the population of our mental institutions. Nor does it lie in such generalized statements as, "Everybody is neurotic." The woeful lack of adequate prevalence or incidence figures on mental and emotional illness today stands as the single greatest hurdle in scientifically determining degree of communicability.

That is why Dr. John Gordon, professor of epidemiology at Harvard, had insisted that "psychiatrists who are trained in epidemiological laboratory methods represent one of our critical needs. [Epidemiology is the science of relating the various factors that determine the frequency and distribution of a disease.]

"If the thoroughness of laboratory method can produce principles for reducing the incidence of mental and emotional sickness, then the door will be open for a grand-scale effort in preventive medicine. Through that door, more of the mentally ill could then pass as cured, and better health might come into view for even 'normal' people who are beset by the growingly complex stresses of modern civilization."

Dr. Gordon's assessment points to a stress complexity that links medicine to a little-appreciated factor in personal well-being: the spiritual health of the patient.

1. How Deadly the Thought, Golin M, *JAMA,* Apr 13, 1957.

2. Is Neurosis Catching?, Golin M, *Charm* magazine, Apr 1959.

Near Life, Near Death, Near God: Devout Impacts and Medicine

Twenty-six-year old Stanley Wisniewski, Jr. was like Lazarus, a man risen from the dead. Just before Christmas of 1954, while at work in the X-ray room at Lutheran Deaconess Hospital in Chicago, he collapsed. His heart had apparently stopped. There was no perceptible pulse.

A doctor quickly cut open the chest cavity with a pocket knife, and after two and a half hours of massage and drugs Wisniewski's heartbeat returned to normal. Newspapers all over the world carried the story, and clinical details were related in *The Journal of the American Medical Association* in 1956 by three participating physicians.

That was the year I was appointed an assistant editor at *JAMA* to "humanize" the publication's 72 years of largely clinical/scientific content (see "Medical Politics" following this chapter.) Editor Austin E. Smith, MD, and I concluded that doing so, in a new editorial department to be named "Medicine at Work," would relate in magazine-style journalism how individuals and organizations outside of medicine work with physicians to approach and maybe help solve major health problems.

For the next three and a half years, I did just that—researching, reporting, writing, and editing 29 *JAMA* papers. These explored such "Medicine at Work" topics as hypnosis, aging, alcoholism, suicide, serendipity in medicine, disaster heroism, and the communicability of neurosis.

They were not mere 500- to 1,500-word news features, but highly readable and incisive investigative reports. Each progressed from a typical 28,000-word first draft to a 4,000- to 6,500-word on-target final product comparable to the research and preparation for *JAMA*'s scientific papers.

In routinely reviewing recent *Journal* papers, I was struck by obvious but unanswered questions in the case of Stanley Wisniewski: Why did he stop breathing? More importantly, why did he survive apparent death for so long? Why did the physicians who attended him not immediately seek, or at least offer, an explanation of the phenomenon? Why?

None of the doctors at AMA could suggest meaningful reasons, although a few noted that brief cessation of breathing during a surgical procedure was not unusual. But for two and a half hours?

So I telephoned each of the three authors of the *JAMA* paper. Two were reluctant to discuss the matter. But the third, C. David Brown, MD, told me after a brief pause, "We did ignore reporting a significant fact: During those crucial two and a half hours, everyone within sight of the victim—nurses, doctors, technicians—was praying, some audibly.[6]

"I was going to mention this in the *JAMA* report, but decided perhaps it was not appropriate in a medical journal. Actually, we felt we were getting some guidance."

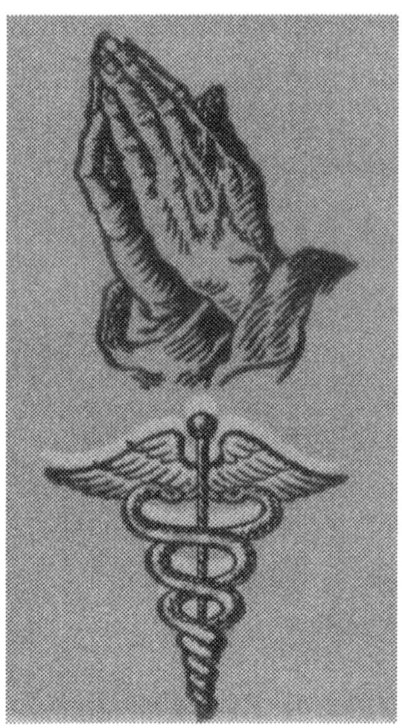

Here was the crux of a significant paper for "Medicine at Work."[6] But the story seemed to cry for much more than a crux. Over three weeks, I wrote and phoned healthcare organizations, medical societies, and religious organizations as well as their members and practitioners, to plumb significant parallels to the Wisniewski experience that were not mere rumors or hearsay.

In that quest, I met with a circuit-riding ordained minister, who also happened to be a licensed physician, making his rounds in rural North Carolina. I interviewed rabbis, like Dr. Henry Raphael Gold of New York, who had become practicing psychiatrists. So have several Catholic priests. One was Jerome Hayden, a Benedictine monk who held doctorates in philosophy and medicine, was teaching psychiatry at a hospital in Washington, DC and seeing patients every day.

A unique service was evolving at the (Protestant) Marble Collegiate Church in New York City, where Dr. Norman Vincent Peale had a full-time staff of psychiatrists, psychologists, and ministers offering a "team approach" to all who seek help. I found that medicine and religion were drawing together more closely than ever before.

Of the 7,000 hospitals in the United States, 1,100 had some religious affiliation and a large proportion of the remainder were ministering to the spiritual needs of their patients. In 35 hospitals clergymen and seminary students received pastoral training in actual contact with the sick and dying.

The Texas Medical Center not only had a program for training ministerial students from five Texas theological schools, but also offered courses in religion for medical students, "to help them learn about the resources the church can offer them in their practice."

The University of Chicago set a precedent when it appointed Granger Westberg, a former hospital chaplain with a D.D. but no M.D., associate professor of religion *and* medicine. Departing was that old line about the minister walking in while the doctor walked out.

When distinguished physicians and clergy of the three major faiths met at the New York Hospital-Cornell Medical Center to discuss the role of religion in healing, their viewpoints were so overlapping that at times the audience seemed to wonder who were the doctors and who were the pastors. It is worth noting, however, that none went so far as to credit "divine intervention" for a successful medical or surgical procedure.

One might suspect that a reluctance of doctors to credit prayer as a factor in a patient's unlikely recovery, as in the case of Stanley Wisniewski in Chicago, might portray them as parties to faith healing. In fact, there was little or no such reluctance. Just the opposite.

This could be because doctors did not wish to be aligned with charlatans in the health field. While unified in their goal of helping patients, ethical physicians and clergy also are firmly allied against "faith healers" who promise miracles. They agreed at the conference that these flamboyant cultists were exploiting the wishful thinking of the ill-informed, sometimes causing needless deaths through delay or abandon-ment of medical care.

For six years the Rev. Carroll Stegall, Jr., a Presbyterian minister from Atlanta GA, had interviewed scores of invalids before and after they lined up at healing campaigns. He reported, "I never saw a vestige of physical change. Not a single so-called healer had submitted one of his alleged cures to medical examination." Yet the religious quacks were collecting millions of dollars from radio, television, and tent shows.

In my three weeks of interviews with doctors and nurses, many were so eager to tell their experiences with patients who were attributing quick recovery at least partly to the prayers or good wishes of loved ones that at times it became necessary to cut short the interviews in order to meet writing deadlines. The finished *JAMA* paper was titled, "Near Life, Near Death, Near God."[2]

Is it unusual to hear devoutness expressed by a physician? Not if you note these typical past comments which, incidentally, could also benefit individuals who extend good wishes (God's wishes) to a patient even though they may not be active in an established religion:

—Dr. Claude E. Forkner, professor of clinical medicine at Cornell University Medical College:" Very often we do not know what it is that brings about the recovery of the patient. I am sure that faith is often a most important factor."

—Dr. Elmer Hess, former president of the American Medical Association: "The doctor has to be a person with firm convictions concerning a Creator. I don't care whether he is Catholic, Protestant, or Jew, so long as he believes in a Power greater than all the instruments of science at his command."

—Dr. Wyatt Norvell of the Kentucky Rural Health Council: "It is impossible to figure out the human body without taking into consideration a Supreme Being."

It was not a theologian but a physician, Sir William Osler, who once said, "Nothing in life is more wonderful than faith—the one great moving force we can neither weigh in the balance nor test in the crucible."

Years later, Dr. C. David Brown, who first told about that Chicago patient whose heart had stopped, finally did theorize clinically how the man was able to survive without a discernable pulse for two and a half hours. While not minimizing the prayer vigil, Dr. Brown believes that undetected blood circulation during that time was adequate to protect the brain from damage.[3]

Medical Politics That Led to a JAMA Revolution

When I walked into the office of *JAMA* editor Dr. Austin Smith on August 20, 1956 for a scheduled 15-minute job interview, little did I realize it would be an entrance to what had been a roiling world of medical politics. Nor did either of us suspect that the interview, stretching to an energized four-hour conference, would revolutionize the way America's leading medical journal shows its face to hundreds of thousands of physicians.

The first five minutes comprised introductions—his background not in medical journalism but as an AMA staff secretary on drug studies, mine as a Chicago City News Bureau investigative reporter and editor. Why was the interview taking place?

For me, because after 12 years at CNB I wanted a broader role and better pay in journalism. For Dr. Smith, because of a passion to forge his own path for *JAMA* as successor to the brilliant, oratorical, dominating Dr. Morris Fishbein . After 25 years in the editor's office, Dr. Fishbein was finally forced out by medical politics in 1949.[1]

The "Fishbeinectomy"[2] ended a long campaign by AMA delegates who had chafed at his taking over their policy-making role. They were determined that no future power like him would occupy the *JAMA* editor's chair. In selecting Dr. Smith to succeed Dr. Fishbein, the AMA could not have settled on a more mirror-opposite choice. Where the ego-driven Fishbein was flamboyant and savvy in medical politics, Smith was studious, apolitical and self-effacing.

The next allotted 10 minutes of interview cascaded out of control as Dr. Smith and I—though never having met before—began to play against one another's ideas for a new feature of the *Journal* to be called "Medicine at Work." It would embody his view of a societal thrust for physician readers. The section would for the first time in its 72-year history provide a real-world counterweight to editorial content that had focused almost entirely on significant but dryly written clinical, scientific, and medical education reports.

After our first hour, at 11 a.m., Dr. Smith had cleared his desk, making room for an exchange of views buttressed by scribbled proposals for deeply researched papers (rather than typically briefer feature articles) that could be read easily. The procedure was for him to suggest general topics and sources that would illustrate doctors' cooperative activities with such nonphysicians as rescue squads (something Dr. Smith had experienced during his ER residency at Bellevue Hospital in New York), civil defense workers, safety experts. My input elaborated on the ideas and included strings of other sources that might flesh out the 5,000- to 6,000-word comprehensive papers.

By noon, as we excitedly were laying out an editorial blueprint for "Medicine at Work," Dr.Smith instructed his secretaries to hold all calls and schedule current appointments for late afternoon. They brought in sandwiches and soft drinks while we worked.

Here was the soft-spoken medical scientist, wearing a Brooks Brothers suit and spit-shine shoes, in an animated jam session with a whooped up scruffy newsman shod in Hush Puppies and clad in a reversible corduroy sports jacket with leather elbow patches. Apparel we had in common were crisp white shirts and bright neckties. The office secretaries surreptitiously peeked in now and then to report back to other staff employees on the unprecedented scene.

At one o'clock Dr. Smith asked if I was willing to begin work immediately, not to report brief feature items, but as *JAMA*'s first-ever nonphysician assistant editor. A sudden start would not be feasible, I explained, because I first needed to complete a City News Bureau assignment directing local coverage of the Democratic presidential nominating convention at the city's International Amphitheater. We agreed that I'd begin in 10 days.

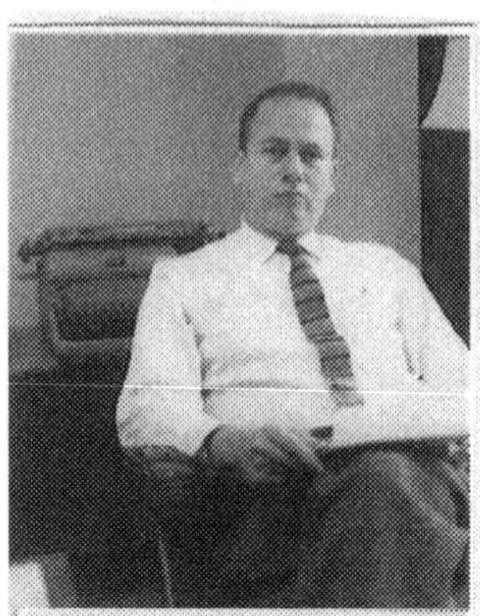

Author as assistant editor of *Journal American Medical Association.* First nonphysician to hold post in 73-year history of *JAMA.*

Also agreed was that while I would alert Dr. Smith in advance of each paper being prepared and seek his advice on some medical sources, he would not edit the product without my consent. (In fact, not once did he wield his blue pencil, even for a single word; self-editing was a rigorous burden to which I had gown accustomed.) Conditioned to 12 years of writing my own news and feature stories anonymously, I desired no byline.

But after one-third of my 29 papers[4] had appeared in *JAMA,* Dr Smith insisted on name attribution. The first paper,[5] on how little towns get good doctors, was a fulfillment of many a journalist's dream: pickup for publication in *The Reader's Digest,* which repeated the honor with another "Medicine at Work" paper* nine months later.[6]

By the time Dr. Smith and I left *JAMA* late in 1959, its ground-breaking "Medicine at Work" section had set the stage for dozens of doctors as well as non-physician staff members whose societal-based editorial content today comprises a significant portion of *Journal* reports.

**"Near Life, Near Death, Near God" reached more people than any other paper in the 121-year history of JAMA. It also marked the first time that a professional journal as well as major national magazines had examined the linkage of medicine and religion so comprehensively. Condensed versions alone, led by* The Reader's Digest *and its foreign editions in six languages, went to more than 18 million readers. Reviews in newspapers and other magazines brought thousands of reprint requests to JAMA*

When reprints were exhausted, AMA reformatted the article into a pamphlet and sent copies to every county and state medical society as well as to 50,000 mem-

bers of the clergy from major denominations.[7] *This led to more sermons and generated an echo effect of additional reprint requests from tens of thousands of doctors, their patients, and members of religious congregations.*

Currently no reprints from any publisher are known to exist.

1. The AMA and U.S. Health Policy, Campion F, Chicago Review Press 1984.

2. ibid

3. Personal communication

4. JAMA papers by assistant editor Milton Golin.

5. Bringing Doctors to Main Street, Reader's Digest, Jan 1957.

6. Near Life, Near Death, Near God, Golin M, JAMA, Apr 19, 1957, and Reader's Digest, Sep 1957.

7. AMA Newsletter, Nov. 20, 1957.

Logging an Armed Mutiny in Wartime

Investigative reporting for the JAMA *"Medicine at Work" paper showing mutual impacts of religion and medicine had its origin a decade earlier. It was in the logbook of a journalist on leave, serving as a U.S. Air Force navigator in World War II, Like an of-duty cop attuned to possible lawbreaking, or a retired physician monitoring medical and healthcare developments, his news-oriented mindset dictates that once a reporter always a reporter.*

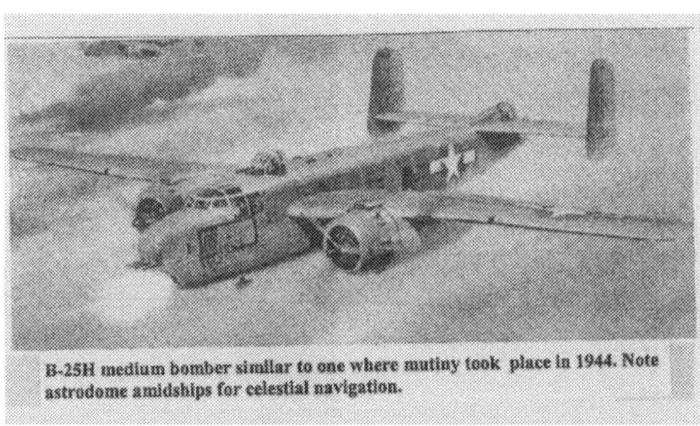
B-25H medium bomber similar to one where mutiny took place in 1944. Note astrodome amidships for celestial navigation.

Periodically recalling the event, I feel on the lam from military police.

Under one viewpoint, I deserve court martial for going against my country in wartime by plotting and leading an armed mutiny—the only one in the history of the U. S. Air Force.[1] In another view, what happened was necessary, to save lives (including mine) and federal property.

By any reasonable measure, the mutiny was neither damnable nor heroic. How then should it be regarded? You be the judge, keeping in mind the events of September 11, 2001. Ask yourself:What would I do if someone aboard my airplane was about to kill me?

One of today's electronic marvels is the Global Positioning Satellites system that informs people and machines exactly where they are. But in the pre-GPS era, transoceanic navigators had to rely heavily on measured sightings of stars and other heavenly bodies to steer thousands of warplanes to combat zones worldwide.

For twin-engine medium bombers—B-25s and B-26s—plying the southern route to combat bases in Britain, Africa, and Asia—the only way to get there in fall or winter was via Ascension Island in the South Atlantic. If crews could not trust the navigator's "fixes," they'd crash in fuel-depleted planes before reaching the island.

The urgent need for rebellion arose Sept. 3, 1944 on my eighth ferrying mission as navigator for the Air Transport Command (ATC).[2] After a dawn routing and weather briefing at Natal, Brazil for crew members, I calibrated the compass of the B-25H (Serial No. 43–5478)* for deviation and variation (correcting magnetic north to true north based on our Brazilian location).

Then I adjusted my chronometer from the vital WWV radio time signal out of Greenwich, England. Departure would be for the longest leg in our India[3] destination: to volcanic-rock Ascension Island, a tiny and isolated spot 1,433 miles east on the map of the South Atlantic. Log entry No. 2.

I squeezed against the tiny desk behind the pilot, piling onto it aeronautical charts, logbook, current almanac, parallel lines ruler, protractor, and related instruments. On the floor I gently laid the bubble laid the bubble octant. I would use it for celestial sightings while standing on a stool in the hemispherical Plexiglas astrodome amidships.

A machine gun emplacement had been removed from the dome to make room for navigation. Wedged next to me, behind the co-pilot, sat the flight engineer, a staff sergeant doubling as radio operator with his own instrument panel.

At 0905 Zulu or GMT (Greenwich Mean Time) on September 3, 1944, we took off along the designated 95-degree course—or so I thought when I wrote the heading on a slip of paper and handed it up to the cockpit as a reminder of the pilot's flight plan. Five minutes later, the compass was edging toward 60 degrees—northeasterly instead of easterly. This was a critical log note.[2]We were barreling toward North Africa, not Ascension Island!

"What are you doing?" I shouted. "The heading is 95." Pilot and co-pilot didn't stir. Then I remembered they could not hear me over the notorious engine noise of the B-25*—such high-decibel not being a great problem in the other planes I had ferried. I flipped on the intercom and said in a normal voice, "Navigator here. The assigned heading starts at 95, not 60. Didn't you hear that at the briefing?"

Even as I spoke, I recalled not having seen the pilot, First Lieut. Jack David, at the briefing, although others of the crew were there, including the co-pilot, Second Lieut. Robert Porterfield.

* The B-25's claim to fame occurred on April 18, 1942 when sixteen B-25s led by Col. James Doolittle took off from The aircraft carrier *Hornet* for a surprise bombardment of Tokyo.

That's OK, Red," David replied. "I know what I'm doing. We'll get there."

"Were you at the briefing?" I asked again. "Because if you were not, we are heading for deep trouble. Change course to 100 degrees until we can straighten this out." My comment and time, 0916, were duly noted.[3]

David did not answer. The compass steadied at 61 degrees. "Lieutenant, this is not the way to Ascension Island," I said. "Change course to 100 or turn back now. Do you copy? Over."

"Yes, I copy. How about getting on that drift meter for a ground speed? Then we can figure ETA [estimated time of arrival]"

"ETA where? The direction you're heading, it won't be to Ascension. Where do you think you *are* going?" The logged time was now 0921 and I was becoming more than a little worried.

"I'm heading directly to Accra," he replied "Save us a whole day. Who needs Ascension?"

Accra, a shoreline airbase of the nation named Gold Coast, was to be our *next* refueling stop after Ascension. Accra is 1,351 miles northeast of Ascension Island, about halfway to our final destination, Karachi, India. I went on:

"Look, you *know* we can't make it that far, even with these extra fuel tanks. Where'd you ever get that idea? At this rate, we'll go down for sure. Please, change course to 105."

"Just relax, Red. If the fuel looks low at the Ascension landfall, we can still get there."

Landfall is the point on one's course where the pilot makes a 90-degree turn—left or right—to reach destination via its sighting or its radio beacon. The flight navigator's goal is to minimize mileage from the turning point or—better yet—eliminate the need for a landfall by periodically fine-tuning the compass heading for direct touchdown on the airport runway.

Now seven hours of vital note-taking would begin. I did some quick figuring on my map. Lieut. David's landfall point would be 600 miles north of Ascension,[2x] the spot where we would crash with depleted fuel tanks. The time was

0930 Zulu and the situation was fast becoming desperate. I quickly took a drift-meter reading from the ocean waves below, measured a 25-knot wind from the northwest, computed a ground speed of 200 knots, handed it to the pilot, and this time ordered—not asked:

"Turn this thing around, back to Natal, or change course to 110 degrees. Do it now."

It was 1015 Zulu and David's's response was steady and calm—and biting: "I don't know what those guys taught you in navigation school, but *you* are not flying this jobbie."

Who was this foolhardy guy at the controls? I asked myself. The other crew members might have wondered, too. After all, we had met one another only for the first time a few weeks earlier (on Aug. 3) in Nashville TN when the B-25 arrived from North American Aviation's Kansas City MO production line.[4]

Two of us were in Nashville, that is. The third, Capt. John Rounds, said to be a veteran ferry pilot, failed to appear. For 25 days we waited for him. Finally, word came that Rounds' name had been scratched from the crew list and that Lieut. David, with limited, short-range transoceanic flight experience, would fill in for him.[4]

On Aug. 28 we had taken off for Morrison Field FL, on the first leg of the ferrying mission. So here, collectively alone over the South Atlantic on Sept. 3, this weird pilot was flying us toward our doom. At 180 miles an hour, we were moving off course at the rate of a mile every 20 seconds.

Now I needed to promptly plot several courses of action. This involved notations not in the limited space of the log, but on my aeronautical chart of the South Atlantic The first step was to fix location. Removing the bubble octant from its case, I obtained a sun line-of-position. Coupled with the drift meter reading, the sunline placed us indeed on a tentative straight shot for Accra.

Next, I spun the thin wheels of my E6B computer—not an electronic device, but a handheld, rotating-disks version of a slide rule—to estimate time, place, and fuel consumption for figuring:

- A "first warning" 360 miles out from Natal (two hours) when we could crash at sea. That would occur at 1700 Zulu, about 340 miles southwest of Roberts Field at Monrovia, Liberia.[2xb]
- A second warning (if necessary) 40 minutes later, based on the same or modified information.
- A point of no return [PNR], from which there simply would be no place to land safely. This would be 860 miles out of Natal at 1300 Zulu.[2xb]

- When to enlist the aid (as needed) of the co-pilot and the nearby flight engineer-radioman after inviting them to my map board location, to point out the series of anticipated positions and calculations.
- When and where—by force, if necessary—to achieve a change of course that could bring us to Ascension Island with available fuel. The E6B computer came up with the answer: 563 miles out of Natal at 1600 Zulu.

For the second time on this mission, which originated from my base, the 4th Ferrying Command in Memphis TN, I strapped on my .45 caliber pistol. The first time had been on the flight leg over jungles of British Guinea and French Guinea five days earlier where, briefing officers routinely warned, headhunters lived and fought—and sometimes decapitated intruders.

My chronometer now showed 1105 Zulu, time for the first warning, at approximate position, logged as four degrees south latitude and 30 degrees west longitude. Again I warned: "Lieutenant, you are flying us to our deaths this plane and all on board. I've just computed ground speed, heading, location, and fuel consumption.

There's *no way* we can make it to Accra. You must—must—either turn back now or change course to 115 degrees. You've got to do this right now, or else!"

"Don't threaten me, a superior officer, you bastard. Just do your job." That's all he said, a comment duly noted. Nor did the incident bring comment from co-pilot Porterfield or the flight engineer-radioman, both of whom I could see were listening to the exchange on their intercom headsets.

Reaching for my octant to update our position, I paused a moment to dwell on its cherrywood case. In childish fashion months earlier, I had used a penknife to carve crudely on its cover: "My Name Is Irene." Her name had also been etched in my mind since that August day in 1942 when I dropped out of college and left my job as a City News Bureau police reporter in Chicago in order to could enlist in the Army Air Corps.[5]

Would I ever see her again? Would the rest of the crew ever see their loved ones? Could I prevent my calculated point-of-no-return from becoming a fact? Only if I could quickly bring a course change.

Now it was 1145 Zulu, signifying a second warning, at a recorded position of three and a half degrees south latitude and 28 degrees west longitude: "Look," I said, we're fast reaching our point of no return. Do you want to die like this, in the drink with sharks? I don't. Who does?

"Can't you understand what's happening here? Lieutenant—Jack—for God's sake, bank to a 120 heading or do a complete 180 for return, *right now*. We can still land at Natal in one piece."

The pilot remained silent, scanning the instrument panel, tight-lipped . I gently poked Lieut. Porterfield to see if I was being heard on the intercom. He nodded yes. I motioned for him to join me at the map board.

Bob Porterfield caught David's eye, started to zip down the fly on his flight suit to indicate he needed to pee in the relief tube, undid his co-pilot harness, and stepped over to my map desk after drawing shut the cockpit curtain. Across the aisle, the sergeant (not identified in my flight log) leaned toward us to watch and overhear. I pointed to the times and positions—now and projected—on my map.

They peered at the figures and lines for about a half-minute. "Are you getting all this?" I asked, speaking over the engine roar against ears now without headset covering. Yes, they nodded. "What do you think?" I asked.

"Well," Porterfield whispered loudly close up, "the filed flight plan *does* show Ascension Island, not Accra. So he is in flight plan violation right there.[5] What do you suggest?"

"Stand ready to take over," I replied. "Any minute now. Sergeant, keep a sharp eye on master switches to use in case David decides quickly to throw me off balance or alert Natal radar to what I'm going to do."

Neither man asked what I would do. They just nodded. Porterfield lingered, then added: "When you said we would not make it to Ascension on this course, I asked David if he was sure about the heading. He said absolutely, he was positive. Now I can see he was dead wrong."

"But why?" I asked. "What's his reasoning? Did you try to talk him into turning right?"

Anxious to return to the cockpit, Porterfield replied quickly, "David says he skipped our briefing so he could be at another one with a flight school pal copiloting a longer-range B-17 to Accra. He seemed determined to stay on his heading, and he was in command. At the time, I didn't know what to do."

Porterfield broke off, hurriedly turning toward the cockpit. But not before I had gathered further from our shouted mouth-to-ear conversation that Lieut. David and his B-17 pal somehow "agreed" that, with forecast favorable tail winds of 40 knots, the B-25 could also make it to Accra nonstop—for a buddy-buddy drink at the officers club bar, to compare notes on the ocean journey.

They apparently had concluded that if "worse came to worst" on fuel consumption, David could still veer south halfway to Accra for a landing at Ascension. Shrewd thinking? No, it was lethal hope.

The four-engine B-17 is faster and has a larger fuel capacity than the B-25 for a nonstop, 2,230-mile flight to Accra. Certainly, David should have known this but decided to ignore it.

The time had now reached 1205 Zulu. I unsnapped the gun holster at my side. Position as noted in the log was three degrees south latitude, 25 degrees west longitude. Rising from my seat and moving toward the cockpit again, I unholstered the .45 caliber pistol and raised it slowly to the back of David's neck.

"That's my sidearm you feel. This is it, Jack. Make the turn now or I'll pull the trigger. Do it now! Bank to 130 degrees." I was 23 years old and reluctantly taking command.

Without moving his head, the pilot darted his bulged eyes sideways at Lieut. Porterfield. Beads of sweat collected on his neck near the gun muzzle. The co-pilot busied himself by scanning the control panel gauges, studiously avoiding David's eyes.

After about 20 seconds—it seemed like an eternity—the pilot's face broke out in a wide grin.

"Holy shit, Red, you weren't kidding, were you?"

Three pairs of eyes watched his hands intently, to detect any sudden movement toward either triggering an alarm or plunging the plane into a distractive descent. In anticipation of diving, co-pilot Porterfield clasped the control column tightly, his knuckles white like his face.

Gently, the plane banked. The compass edged to 130 degrees. "OK, we're on track." said David. "Get me an ETA."

I continued to hold the pistol up, but away from his neck, for fully one minute, then holstered it. The course held steady under clear skies as I returned to the drift meter for an ocean-waves reading. Then I computed ground speed for an ETA, neatly wrote the figures on a scrap of paper, and handed it up. The ordeal was almost over—almost, because there was only my estimate (from the handheld E6B calculator) of fuel consumption, that we'd make it to Ascension Island.

What had we just done? No, what had *I* done? This was mutiny, armed insurrection against the command pilot. Not mere insubordination. We all knew what this could mean for me in wartime: a court martial conviction punishable by execution.

Sure, there were serious charges against the pilot: filing a false flight plan, failing to adhere to it, refusing to attend a required briefing, endangering the lives of Air Corps personnel and of federal property, the B-25.

Except for dodging a 30-minute thunderstorm, the rest of the flight proceeded smoothly—and except for a remaining major concern: Did we have enough fuel? I shot another sunline, computed a 25-knot tailwind, handed up two more ground speeds and ETAs, and started nibbling at a C-ration candy bar.

Fuel tank gauges were edging toward empty. By 1700, roughly a half-hour to go, we picked up an Ascension Island radio signal—and in five minutes confirmed that it was not a spurious transmission for the surfaced German submarine known to have tried luring fuel-shy warplanes into destruction at sea. I recognized the voice a few seconds later as definitely from the control tower.

The co-pilot and pilot conversed sparingly, neither of them speaking to me. The fuel gauges were now *at* empty. When informed of this, the control tower operator directed a straight-in touchdown, rather than follow an approach pattern. Landing was at 1735 in poor visibility as the B-25 rumbled over the expected mid-runway bump, an unavoidable relic of difficult construction on the lava-rock island.

More log-entries: ETA was two minutes late, the landfall 20 miles left of my estimation—not too bad considering the circumstances. Fuel on board was a mere 20 gallons, a close call indeed.

(Ironically, today Ascension Island serves as one of a pattern of global monitoring stations that assure the accuracy of the 28-satellite global positioning system.)

At the debriefing, each of us expected that one or more of the others would spill the beans, say what had happened en route, explain arriving an hour later than it usually takes from Natal. The debriefing officer did not ask what took so long, merely noted my report of en route weather conditions. None of us spoke up. We did not answer unasked questions. It was as if nothing unusual had occurred.

But an hour after the landing, the gun-slinging scene at the cockpit began replaying itself in my mind. There was no question that I did what I had to do. But other questions were nagging:

Had I been serious in my threat? Was I bluffing? Would I really have fired the pistol?—to kill or wound the pilot? In my Ascension Island sleeping quarters that night, I was able to answer only the first two questions. I had not been bluffing; the threat had been life-threateningly serious.

In the weeks that followed, other questions hung tentatively—except for the conviction that I could not have killed the pilot. Murder is not in me.

Today I can only speculate whether my mindset at the cockpit would have sent a bullet into Lieut. David's foot on the rudder pedal or a hand on the controls or through an overhead or Plexiglas side panel (at 9,000-foot altitude, the plane's interior was safely unpressurized.}

What transpired after the debriefing, however, is another story. That's how rumors start—in this case, as we and others would learn later, a far-reaching rumor of mutiny that may very well persist to this day.

But it was more than a rumor. Unlike today's typical urban legend, in which a possible event is told as reality, this happening is documented by navigation log entries and buttressed by en route map notations. In the months that followed the incident, I had heard versions of the mutiny from:

- An Air Transport Command briefing in Shanghai.
- A ferrying pilot in Townsville, Australia.
- Two navigators at an officers' club in Casablanca.
- Two fellow meteorology/navigation briefing officers when I was assigned to Himalayan "Hump" duty in Burma.
- A China-Burma-India Veterans Association historian in Nacogdoches, Texas.

If the pilot had thought of pressing charges, I came to believe he feared the consequences for himself. And perhaps, I thought, the co-pilot and the sergeant felt the same way about their involvement.

At 0735 the next day, September 4, 1944, with refueling and maintenance complete, and briefed for weather and heading, we took off for Accra. The flight was nearly as long as the previous day's—1,351 miles. Although the weather was rougher, I was able to shoot two sunlines that fixed with radio signals from West Africa. ETA was good, three minutes late. Dead reckoning was poor.

After Accra, there were seven more flight legs before delivery of the B-25 in Karachi . During that time, the pilot said not one word to me, nor I to him. His navigation questions were relayed via co-pilot Porterfield: What heading? What ground speed? What ETA?

Not that the remaining seven flight legs were uneventful. Along the 650-miles from Accra to Kano, Nigeria, the gyroscope on the artificial horizon stopped working, and during the same day's 275-mile trip to Maidugari, Nigeria the command radio equipment failed. Fortunately, weather in both cases was clear enough for dead reckoning navigation by land marks. Each of my ETAs was only one minute off.

On the 750-mile leg next day, September 6, to El Fasher in Egyptian Sudan, the pilot decided abruptly to drop to a 3,000-foot altitude from 7,000 feet and stray about 40 miles north of course to view Lake Chad. He then dived the plane to 200 feet to buzz the lake, a refuge for many thirsty animal species and their predators.[5]

Close up, we could see perhaps a thousand or more creatures scattering in panic at the roar of the B-25's engines. David's unexpected descent and reckless buzzing of Africa's most precious natural animal refuge seemed to me consistent with his dangerously impulsive course from Natal, Brazil.

By the time we reached Karachi on September 9,[6] with refueling stops at Khartoum in the Sudan, Aden in Arabia, and Masirah Island off Oman, Porterfield, David, and the staff sergeant had become more sociable.

They speculated on their next ferrying mission, perhaps to bases in Australia or Scotland.

Wordlessness between Lieut. David and me continued, even as I issued $100 vouchers to each crew member in Karachi for their minimum four hours per month overseas extra flight pay. Routinely, these payments were an assigned duty of every ATC navigator who ferried crews, possibly because only he could certify their in-air foreign time accurately from entries in his log.

After 36 hours of rest in Karachi, all four of us boarded a C-47 cargo plane for return to the States—as passengers, not as crew. By the time of a refueling stop at Cairo, Egypt, tenseness with Lieut. David had eased—to the point where he and I and Lieut. Porterfield were posing for a desert cameraman at the Pyramids.[3x]

Three months later, on another ferrying trip, I recognized a new briefing officer at Ascension Island as a former Wright College classmate in Chicago, Eric Asplundh. Our offhand conversation included something like this:

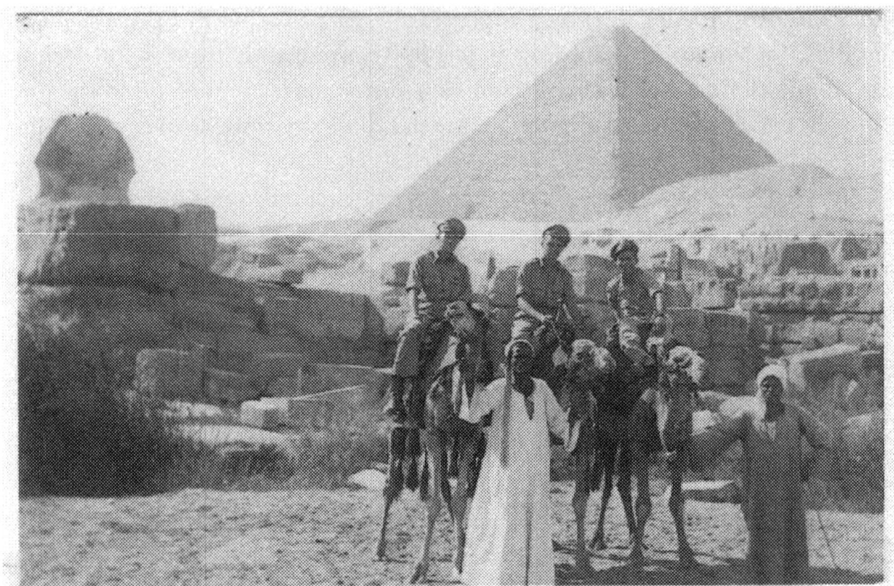

After delivering mutiny-punctuated ferrying mission of B-25 bomber to India air base, crew poses for desert photographer at Pyramid en route back to U.S. Left to right are author-navigator Milton Golin, co-pilot Robert Porterfield, and pilot Jack David.

"Eric, ever hear about some navigator taking over a flight here from Brazil because the pilot refused to follow the assigned compass heading?"

"Sure. Not only that, I heard he held a gun to the pilot's head to get him to change course."

"Then what?"

"I never found out. The plane, a medium bomber, is supposed to have landed here OK, but nobody seems to know who the guys were or what finally happened to them."

After my discharge from the Army Air Corps at Fort Sheridan near Chicago in February of 1946, I pondered frequently about that scary event over the South Atlantic—why it remained untold for so long.

What does the record show about instances of mutiny in the Air Force?

Without mentioning my experience, I posed that question early in March 2001 to three Pentagon officials:

Air Force historian Dr. Richard P. Hallion; Dr. Lawrence J. Delaney, the Air Force chief information officer; and the Air Force judge advocate general.[7]

One response documented three Air Force mutinies, all occurring in World War II and each involving racial tensions—Negro (the operative word then) troops in Texas rebelling at unfair or cruel demands of white officers. None of those mutinies involved use of weapons.[8] Not surprisingly, there was no mention of ours over the South Atlantic.

Another response, from James Russell, a civilian attorney for the Air Force who is associate chief of the Military Justice Division at Bolling Air Force Base in Washington DC, questioned whether a true mutiny had taken place.

"Pulling a pistol on a commander would be a fairly serious thing," he told *Chicago Magazine* writer Robert Kurson. "The charges might be 'assaulting a superior officer' or perhaps 'disobeying an order.' But mutiny takes more than one person in the Articles of War of 1949. In any case, mutiny courts-martial were rare, as were executions."[9]

Russell seems to have overlooked the fact that I had two co-conspirators, the co-pilot and the flight engineer.

Until now, revealing my role as a reluctant mutineer would incriminate not only me but also the other crew members. They would not likely welcome such notoriety, however latter-day. And, for all I know, Lieut. David would also have long wished to forget about that life-threatening standoff in the cockpit. After all, he was as culpable as I, for ignoring an official flight plan.

This is why I have kept silent about details of the episode for more than a half-century. At first, it was a reluctance to face court martial. In later years, though, the secrecy has been motivated by a desire to prevent exposure of an event for which personal guilt remains.

The events of September 11, 2001 leads me to re-evaluate that flight in September 1944. There's probably not an American today who hasn't contemplated what to do on an airplane if he believed his life was being threatened. Many who wouldn't have known how to react on that day in 1944 might have changed their minds by now.

Why am I speaking out now? Because at last I feel no concern for the consequences, come what may. Never mind that what I did resulted in the saving of lives and property. Never mind that, in all likelihood, too much time has elapsed for any military prosecution to succeed.

Yet, the feeling of shame persists. I have felt this way for years, every time there was a patriotic display or parade. It has been a shadow.

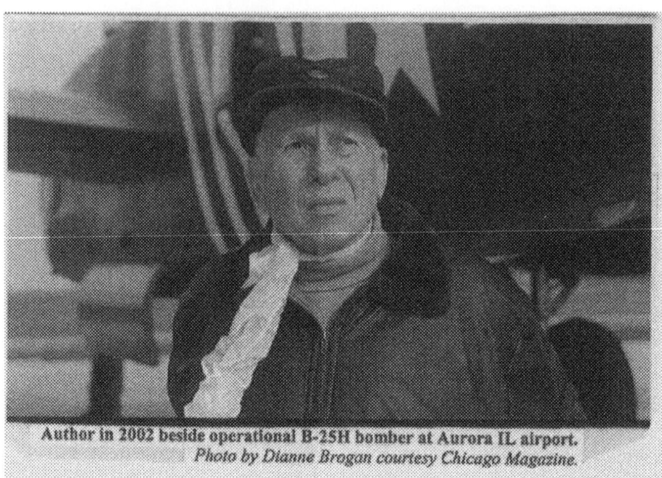
Author in 2002 beside operational B-25H bomber at Aurora IL airport.
Photo by Dianne Brogan courtesy Chicago Magazine.

How can I be proud of having led an armed insurrection while other Americans were giving and risking their lives? The answer is: I am not.

For the navigator, the mutiny was a prelude to his return as a reporter where, on Chicago's city hall beat, he encountered an unanswered question about a deadly bit of American history

1. Letters to and from U.S. Air Force historian P. Hallion, archivist Archie Difante, and historical research commander Col. Carol S. Sikes.

2. Air Navigation log of Lieut. Milton Golin.

3. World map of Lieut. Golin's ATC missions.

4. ibid. navigation log.

5. ibid.

6. ibid.

7. See footnote 1.

8. ibid.

9. A Mutiny of One, Kurson R, *Chicago* magazine, June 2002.

Finding Theodore Roosevelt's Savior

News is not necessarily something that only occurs today or yesterday. It can also be a significant happening from years ago that had hardly or ever been fully told.

As a reporter covering Chicago's city hall in 1950, my eye caught a routine aldermanic vote that "memorialized" Frank Bukovsky for "laudable activity" on Oct. 14, 1912. When I asked for more information, clerks said that he and his neighbors could relate a fuller story involving an assassination attempt at a political rally in Milwaukee.

It was easy enough locating Bukovsky. Harder was interviewing him and his wife Marie in their southwest side Bohemian neighborhood. They knew only limited English. Nearby friends stepped in to translate, and fascinating story elements emerged [1] ("Chicago's Forgotten Hero," in the March 1951 issue of *Coronet,* was my first article sale to a national magazine.)

Frank recalled running up the three flights of stairs to his flat to show Marie the newspaper headline:

"T. R. at Milwaukee Auditorium Tonight." The initials, he explained, were for Theodore Roosevelt, who as President six years earlier had signed papers enabling entry of the Bukovskys into the U. S. "I must go to see him," he told Marie.

What happened next included Frank's words in our interview plus details gathered later from Milwaukee and New York City newspapers:

Frank was downtown early, outside the Gilpatrick Hotel. He could almost touch the car that was to take Teddy from the hotel to the auditorium a few blocks away, where several thousand people were waiting for him. The former President stepped into the car and stood on the back seat, grinning and waving his black slouch hat to the smiling crowd—nothing at all like in native Bohemia, where soldiers with rifles guarded the emperor in the passing coach.

It was then that Frank Bukovsky noticed the wild-eyed man standing next to him. Suddenly the man reached inside his coat and pulled a revolver. The next moment he was taking aim at Roosevelt's heart—a heart only seven feet away. As the gun went off with a roar, Frank slammed his hand against the man's right arm. Then he knocked him to the ground to stop more shooting.

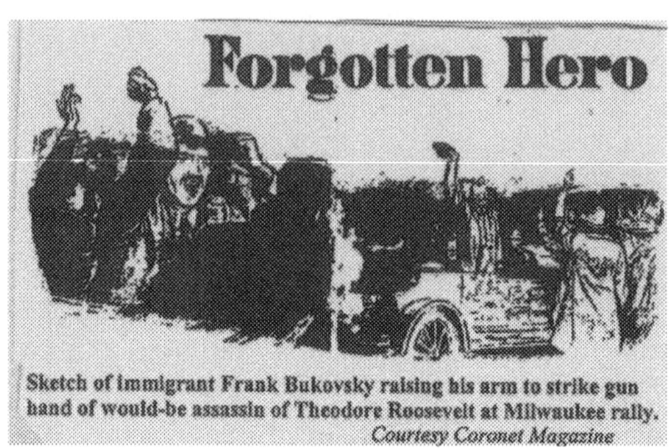
Forgotten Hero

Sketch of immigrant Frank Bukovsky raising his arm to strike gun hand of would-be assassin of Theodore Roosevelt at Milwaukee rally.
Courtesy Coronet Magazine

"Kill him! Kill him!" Frank shouted in English. Then he added in Bohemian, "Kill this crazy man! He shot our great Roosevelt."

The shocked crowd understood only the American words. They thought that Frank, the curly-haired man with the foreign accent, was going to kill Roosevelt. Some of them piled onto Frank as well as on the gunman.

A policeman swung his club on Frank's head. His clothes ripped, his hat smashed, Bukovsky tore himself away and ran home. Next morning, he looked through the newspapers. His name was not mentioned.

The paper said that Elbert Martin, Roosevelt's secretary, had saved his life by snatching the gun from the assassin, John Flammang Schrank. The news account also reported that a man in the crowd had hit Schrank's arm so that the bullet, instead of entering Roosevelt's heart, struck him on the right side of the chest, first passing through 100 pages of his speech.

Roosevelt, shocked and bleeding, made the speech anyway. Later, at the hospital, he remarked: "It takes more than one bullet to kill a Bull Moose."

Three weeks later, Frank Bukovsky voted in his first Presidential election—for Theodore Roosevelt, the "Bull Moose" candidate. He was not perturbed when Woodrow Wilson won. That was democracy.

Years later his idol, Theodore Roosevelt, died. With his wife, three daughters, and a son, Frank Bukovsky moved to Chicago, where he bought a bakery near neighbors from old Bohemia.

The family lost virtually everything in the Depression—the bakery, the home, the bank account—more than $40,000 saved over many years. They did not lose their spirit and faith in their country.

In 1943, Bukovsky read in the newspapers that John Schrank had died in a Wisconsin asylum. And the story of the attempted assassination was revived. A newspaper revealed that Frank Bukovsky had been written up in an old history book as the man who really saved Theodore Roosevelt's life. The book mentioned half a dozen people who actually saw how Frank upset Schrank's aim. But the newspaper also said, despite decades of search by journalists and historians, that Frank could not be found—that he was probably dead.

Reading the last part, he mused: "I was not seeking any notoriety. When new friends would hear him tell what happened back in 1912, they'd ask: No medal, Frank? No reward? Not even a letter—a note from somebody in the Roosevelt family?" No, not even a letter; nothing.

Routinely he would reply, "Do I need any greater reward than my four children—all of them educated, successful, happy? Me, a poor immigrant from Bohemia?"

Frank Bukovsky's warm relationship with his children is a rarity for millions of other families that are torn by an all-too-common addiction: alcoholism. Daring doctors have joined with other groups to help minimize this massive problem.

1. Chicago's Forgotten Hero, Golin M, *Coronet* magazine, March 1951.

Pursuing Alcoholism, Robber of Five Millions Brains

You ride figuratively with 26 terrified children as their school bus careens wildly over the steep and winding road near Ironton, Ohio—and you jump as they jump, in wide-eyed ones and twos, when the bus sways like crazy at every curve. The driver is intoxicated—a problem drinker.

You stand beside the bleary-eyed executive in his locked Manhattan office while he bangs down a rubber stamp facsimile signature which he hopes will ez- cuse him from the scrawl that is a dead giveaway of the shakes. Liquor is his boss.

Smell the breath of that Texas salesman as he stops his car to "fortify" himself with a swig of rum. Catch the Wisconsin logger's wife when he knocks her across the room in bourbon rage. Peek through the apartment window of the San Fran- cisco secretary "staying in with a headache" while she solitarily starts an all-day gin binge.

This is alcoholism, a complex disorder that prompts the unthinking to joke about drunks but can leave families homeless and penniless; a massive medical puzzler which is no less soluble because it also is a major sociological and economic problem; a public cancer that can turn some individuals against themselves but to which others are completely resistant; a blight so singularly human that the Bible warns against it, Shakespeare diagnoses it, and Tennessee Williams builds a prize-winning play around it.

According to a *Journal of the American Medical Association* investigative report[1], drink has taken five million men and women in the United States, taken them as masters take slaves, and new acquisitions are going on at the rate of 200,000 a year. Yet, the disease that lurks in alcohol is a fickle tyrant—choosing, unexplainably, the one drinker out of every 16 over whom it is able to exert complete control.

This is because, in a larger sense, the culprit is not alcohol. It is alcoholism. Oddly enough, the great majority of drinkers cannot acquire this sickness no matter how hard they may try.

One who tried is a New York City physician who, purely in the interest of medical science (for a *JAMA* paper), set out to prove with his own body that alcohol was as addictive as morphine. He loaded the trunk of his car with cases of whisky and drove to an isolated cabin in New England. There, day after day and night after night, he drank and sang and drank. But he was not happy.

For at the end of one solid month of inebriation, when the doctor returned to his office to measure his cravings and physical dependency on alcohol as a drug, only one thing was certain: He did not want to even look at liquor for the rest of his life.[2]

What the experiment did establish (and the proof is not new) was that alcoholism, like cancer, cannot be implanted in simply anyone by physiological means alone. A multiplicity of other conditions are also disease factors. Tests with animals bear this out.

An elephant, for example, is subject to severe stomach cramps if it is exposed to severe cold weather for a prolonged period and will start trumpeting with pain. Its physical hurt plus accompanying psychological stress can be relieved by a large bucket of gin and ginger. But after taking this remedy a few times, the elephant becomes a crafty alcoholic, feigning pain and moaning pitifully for its daily swig.

Cats have been turned into alcoholics by spiking their milk with liquor while placing them in a variety of frustrating situations. In similar tests with rats under nonstress conditions, the rodents were able to take their whisky or leave it.

Alcoholism in man is basically a brain disease—insofar as the brain is a physiologic organ subject to blood changes, a psychological organ subject to mental and emotional stresses, and a sociological organ subject to interpersonal demands and byplay.

Like syphilis, alcoholism at last is being fought out in the open—spotlighted as a disease that responds to treatment, rather than beclouded as an irredeemable moral failing that forever must be condemned in the individual and tolerated in the mass. Who are physician allies in the war against alcoholism? They are clergymen and businessmen, labor leaders and schoolteachers, lawyers and bartenders, policemen and playwrights. And they are the alcoholics themselves.

Every recovered alcoholic is a particularly incisive fighter against his own disorder—more thorough than the ex-tuberculosis patient trying to limit the spread of TB, more effective than the heart attack survivor seeking to defeat cardiac diseases, more influential than the cancer victim hoping to ease the lives of others so stricken.

More than 150,000 alcohol addicts-turned-counselors credit their savior, Alcoholics Anonymous. Their "strength amid weakness" is shown in the successful activities of thousands of AA groups across the nation. Yet, because the organization's therapy tends to help only those who can adjust to the intense group life of its program, many alcoholics are not treatable through this approach. By their very nature, many alcoholics are antisocial.

One New Jersey addict put it this way to his physician: "I don't like to hear other people's troubles at those AA meetings." Yet, Alcoholics Anonymous effectively deals with the sickness. For thousands of victims it is the avenue for a life free from compulsive drinking. Not only in AA but in the efforts of diverse organizations and individuals the disease is fought with vigor:

In New York City, clergymen and judges joined medical leaders as lecturers in courses established at Fordham University for social workers who deal with alcoholics.

In Chicago, the police department has operated a Fellowship Club for the rehabilitation of officers afflicted with alcoholism. Founded in 1954, it is the first organization of its kind, prompting a pattern for police administrators in San Francisco and other cities. Not too long ago no police force would dare admit it had an alcohol addiction problem.

In California, a 10% liquor license fee increase was helping to finance eight alcoholism rehabilitation clinics on a shared-cost basis with communities. (According to a *JAMA* paper, "For reasons not yet fully determined, more alcoholics per capita have been reported in San Francisco than in any other American city. The incidence there was nearly four times that of the over-all U.S. rate.

What stands out in every community battle against alcoholism is the judgment of the physician. It is he or she who decides when, if, and how tranquilizers, vitamins, and abstinence-training drugs shall be used—also guiding and observing, researching and coordinating, evaluating and mobilizing, sympathizing and debunking, inspiring and persuading.

The skilled doctor is defending patients from abuse, pioneering new concepts, trying to do a job of preventive medicine. The rub is that not enough physicians are doing this. There are still many doctors who shun the problem drinker as a patient.

At the same time, however, thousands more—particularly primary care physicians—are realizing that the burden of treating an alcoholic no longer need be borne by them alone, that there are growing numbers of medical and nonmedical resources available to help them in the task. And where community resources are not available, some physicians have taken the initiative to organize appropriate services.

One reason that alcoholism is such a difficult disease is that its exciting agent is a two-faced creature—a liquid that holds both good and evil, that can provide release or can enslave. This mysterious and sometimes unpredictable catalyst of the brain has some therapeutic value as well as harmful effects.

In moderate doses it can offer the noncompulsive drinker needed relaxation from the cares of the day, help relive the pain of rheumatoid arthritis, stimulate the appetite, aid digestion, and help relieve some symptoms of the common cold (by providing warmth and comfort, inducing drowsiness, and creating desire for rest.) Imbibed in moderation, it also has been shown to improve cardiac function.

The "good" face of alcohol sometimes may be difficult to recognize, particularly by those well-meaning persons who advocate prohibition as the only solution to "the evils of drink" The repeal of Prohibition in the 1930s ended an era in which alcoholics and controlled drinkers alike experienced rotgut suffering amid an inevitable lawlessness that extended beyond the speakeasy.

While alcohol is a depressant, in small amounts it might also improve awareness. In a surprising case cited in a *JAMA* [3], a casual imbiber caught a television crew and audience off guard in a large city. According to script, the man was supposed to illustrate the dangers of alcohol by first operating a driver testing machine in a sober condition and then with two drinks under his belt.

But it didn't work out that way. At the start, the subject was nervous in a strange situation and he scored badly. He did well after the drinks. Television cameras recorded the experiment faithfully, much to the puzzlement and frustration of the show's producer, who felt right then that it was he who needed a drink.

Had the drinking man in the studio been driving a real automobile instead of operating a stationary testing device, his "score" might have been tragic. The chief danger in really driving after a few drinks is the soaring confidence which leads to taking chances.

Other excerpts from the *JAMA* report, "Facts on Alcohol and Alcoholism"[4] include:

- By gradually consuming half a highball or three quarters of a can of beer every hour, the "average" adult can drink 24 hours a day without becoming intoxicated. (This is the average rate alcohol oxidation by the human liver—and of course no individual is average.)
- As little as 0.04 of alcohol in the blood may reduce visual acuity as much as the wearing of dark glasses after sundown.

- For each of the estimated five million alcoholics in the U.S., another four persons—family, employer, friends—are closely affected, making a total of 25 million people involved intimately in the problem today.
- Alcoholics are extraordinarily rare among observant Jews. The reason is not known for certain, but one recurrent theory is that a dignified respect for wines at closely knit family rituals during childhood may be a factor.
- A "hybrid" type of alcoholic, sometimes called the superalcoholic, limits his drinking to such poisons as witch hazel, rubbing alcohol, antifreeze, and "canned heat." These "supers" deny trying to kill themselves, insisting that they drink the potent stuff because conventional liquors are too tame.
- The bill for alcoholism in the United States was estimated at more than one billion dollars a year—in work time lost, accidents, reduced and spoiled work output, and welfare payments to families of nonworking alcoholics. This is a direct economic cost only, and does not cover crime attributable to the disorder nor such immeasurable losses as the human misery in interpersonal crises, broken homes, warped personalities, and dulling of minds.

New concepts as to the causes of alcoholism are being explored and collated with research findings in an effort to find a way to prevent the disease—or at least spot it in potential victims at an early age, when preventive measures might be attempted. One medical researcher in the subject, Dr. Giorgio Lolli of New York City, has called alcoholism "a disorder of the love disposition" originating in childhood frustrations.

His thesis might be reflected in widespread current binge drinking among college and even high school and younger students. That trend stands in sharp contrast to the therapeutic activities of other teens and pre-teenagers, notably in Phoenix, Arizona. Read on.

1. "Robber of Five Million Brains," Golin M, *JAMA,* Jul 19, 1958, Vol. 167 No.12, pp. 1496–1502.

2. ibid.

3. ibid.

4. ibid.

Don't Call Them Baby-Sitters

One morning in May 1959, a surprising phone call came from a Saturday Evening Post *editor who had read my stories on Frank Bukovsky and the Louisiana hurricane. He asked if I would be willing, on short deadline, to go to Phoenix, AZ and "vitalize" a rejected manuscript about children stricken with cerebral palsy. He felt that the turned-down story was heart-rending but weak in reader interest.*

I was flabbergasted and flattered because I knew no one at the magazine and never had suggested an article to it, I readily agreed to the assignment. In the midst of 29 interviews, the story began taking an unexpected turn—from dominant sympathy for the stricken kids and toward a dual focus on the plight of CP parents and on praise for a cadre of dedicated young caregivers.

Discussions with the parents revealed that they were being helped dramatically by youths who were specially trained to manage specific medical aspects of the crippling disorder. With deft coaching (via questions rather than directives or suggestions) from Saturday Evening Post *associate editor Arnold Nicholson, I was able to produce a June 20, 1959 cover line story.*

It emphasized the assurance of parents, after years of homebound isolation, that their disabled young children were with competent young caregivers. At the same time, the article pointed up the character-building experience of these skilled teenagers. As rejuvenated, the story thus reached a more meaningful conclusion, piquing the interest of parents and children everywhere, healthy or not[1]*.*

There is nothing deadly about cerebral palsy (although there is plenty of high drama), unless you factor in shortened longevity. Yet, many parents of CP children, unable to escape the burden of care, might consider the seemingly endless months and years of in-home confinement with their children a virtual death sentence. In Phoenix, Arizona some amazing teenagers enliven the scene.

Once a week at a house on a palm-shaded street in Phoenix, Judy Weinmeister calls to monitor her friend Lincoln (Linc) Lynde, aged eight. "Monitor" is her title—Judy is no ordinary baby sitter.

Linc has cerebral palsy, a brain-to-muscle disorder that afflicts 600,000 persons in the United States. For a few hours Judy relieves the Lyndes in their day-in-day-out task of watching over him. She reads to Linc, plays games with him, and manages a limited conversation through his speech difficulty.

Judy is one of 110 young men and women—plus one widowed grandmother—who are certified as Cerebral Palsy Monitors, caring for youngsters who need special help now and then. Thanks to them, a measure of normal living is in sight for more than 1,000 CP families in Central Arizona. For too long, many of these families have isolated themselves, often in the false belief that somehow they are to blame for their children's condition.

"People still hide the youngsters in attics and cellars," says Linc's father, Fred Lynde, Sr., because, as parents, they fail to understand this is not a humiliating result of their own heredity. "I'm not ashamed to take Linc with me anywhere—camping, fishing, down the street for a walk," says Lynde. "People look at him and I know what some of them are thinking as he struggles for words, or flails an arm, or screws up his face."

Lynde's words bring a nod of understanding from Judy, a Camelback High School sophomore who hopes to be a social worker. "Linc is more lovable and easier to handle than the normal children I sit for," she says.

Monitors such as Judy must earn their titles. They absorb instruction from physicians, nurses, therapists, and social workers. They sit on the edge of their chairs in rapt attention, looking at slide films and movies which explain cerebral palsy. Eagerly, they acquire the skill of attaching and removing braces from the legs of a youngster who smiles through his handicap. They know what it means to need help and to give help.

It was just before Christmas of 1957 that several dozen parents of palsied children met at the United Cerebral Palsy office in Phoenix to plan a Santa Claus party. Not until after the formal session did they pour out their problems. Two fathers compared costs of specialized care for their crippled kids. A housewife bemoaned the impossibility of getting away from her apartment in order to work or gain added funds. Several other mothers dreamed aloud about the unreachable luxury of a carefree evening:

"My husband and I haven't been out together, not even to a movie, since our daughter was born eight years ago…"

"Most sitters don't know what cerebral palsy is. They freeze up and say no to our calls when we mention our son's condition…"

"Isn't there some way sitters can be taught to take proper care of our children, so that we might have some relaxation and variety, give our youngsters relief from us?" parents asked.

With the idea thus formally born, Mrs. Alice Carver, an arts and crafts teacher, nurtured it. She lined up talks by a county health nurse and a medical specialist in cerebral palsy. She also scheduled descriptive films and five demonstrations. But what really got the monitors program off the ground was help from the high schools.

When superintendents learned about the extended student education, they passed the word to principals, who discussed the nascent program with school nurses, science-club advisors, and more than 50 career counselors. Announcements went over classroom loudspeakers and in daily bulletins. Suddenly school pride was being put to the test.

The day of the first monitor class, 75 students from seven Phoenix-area high schools showed up in their Sunday best. One demonstration particularly impressed the teenagers. A speech therapist was teaching a cerebral-palsied girl how to blow out a match, so that she might pronounce certain words. Tensely, the fascinated students held fists clenched and jaws ajar—as if to "think" the girl into speaking.

The scene was etched into the mind of Ellen Darland, a senior at Camelback High. Weeks later, during summer vacation, while six-year-old Dennis Mitcham's mother worked days, Ellen monitored the cerebral-palsied boy.

"I was determined that he say the word 'blue,'" Ellen recalls. "Every day I placed a candy wafer at his mouth and promised he could eat it if he kept it between his lips while I counted to ten. That soon brought the first letter in "blue,' and one day he said the whole word. I was so thrilled. We both laughed and laughed. Denny showed me how a handicap can challenge people to help."

One young lady on monitor duty was dwarfed by a 16-year-old boy who was subject to *grand mal* (epilectic) seizures. He suffered an attack on her first evening with him, and she became frightened—but only long enough to remember what to do.

As the youth began to fall, his arms flailing helplessly, she seized him from behind and eased him to the floor, rolling him onto his left side. Swiftly taking a gauze-padded, wooden mixing-spoon handle from her monitor kit, she pushed it firmly but gently between his teeth. When he became quiet, the girl loosened his collar. Then she telephoned the family physician, who advised letting the victim sleep. It went as smoothly as a monitor-course demo.

That illustrates a strict rule for teaching the monitors: Do not give them medical training—only first aid, tips on common-sense child care, and home-nursing routines. "Yes, the monitors know their limitations," says Dr. William La Joie, a specialist in physical rehabilitation. "It is pure joy speaking to those teenagers—watching their enthusiasm, their grasp at every word said, the quiet intenseness. I can actually see those kids soak up a feeling of responsibility."

In what way are CP children afflicted? Cerebral palsy is a general term for a group of disorders caused by injury to the "motor centers" and related areas of the brain. These brain cells function as traffic policemen, directing the muscles in various parts of the body. In a normal person, the signal which converts a thought into action operates almost automatically. But in the cerebral palsied, jumbled signal responses may create a traffic jam.

There is impairment of voluntary muscle control, awkward movements, lack of balance, irregular gait, guttural speech, grimacing, drooling, spasms, or rigidity. But many CPs are acutely aware of the world around them—sounds, smells, tastes, color, touch. A monitor will tell you that they know the number of steps to the schoolhouse, the rustle of a falling leaf, the goodness of home-baked cookies, the beauty of a rain-washed day.

As the monitors learn in their course, cerebral palsy can develop from faulty growth of brain cells before birth, cerebral injury during birth, or brain damage later from head injury or certain severe illnesses. A palsied child may have the I.Q. of a genius—or be classified psychologically as a moron. He or she may be impulsive and unpredictable—or reliable and thoughtful. But no matter what his intellect or personality, the CP child exerts an important influence upon his entire family.

Parents of cerebral-palsied children can select a monitor from names in a special U.C.P. directory, 600 copies of which have been distributed free of charge to their homes. Copies also go to physicians, clinics and hospitals, visiting nurses, parent-teacher groups, nursery schools and kindergartens, the Youth Employment Service, and other health agencies.

Monitors charge the same rates as sitters for normal children, although occasionally a bonus may be forced upon them. Joanne Gerlach, a junior at South Mountain High, remembers the happy expressions of one pair of CP parents when they returned home after a first night out in years. They were so pleased that, after paying Joanne, they showered her with all the coins in a cookie jar.

Experiences such as Joanne's are carried back to school—as reports for English, citizenship, and other classes. Peter McClintock delivered two talks on the monitors to his public-speaking class. Joanne Gerlach helped compile a research theme describing the program. Judythe Schott, a North High sophomore, broughtit up for discussion in biology studies. "Lots of kids see themselves as second-class until they become adults, Judythe tells her classmates, "but monitors have no reason to feel that way."

Why should that be so? Edward J. Stancik, director of student personnel services for the Phoenix Union High School system, offers an explanation: "The monitor program seems to typify the characteristics of opportunity to these young people, the chance to contribute directly—something many teenagers cannot otherwise experience. We see that this is not a vehicle for self-aggrandizement, but of maturing responsibility."

The program also can build better lives, attitudes, and careers. For illustration you need only listen to tall, brown-eyed Deanna Dean, a senior at North High.

"I want to be a social worker, but why do most students rate it so low as a career?" Deanna asks. "I think it is because schools push engineering, math, chemistry, physics, bomb scares. You're told you have to be a walking genius or they'll blow up the world around you. Left out of the future are literature and journalism and civics and law and social work and the arts—some of the directly human vocations.

"Maybe this has something to do with today's juvenile delinquency. Maybe more teenagers need a new outlook. I have a new outlook on just about everything, simply from the monitor course—understanding people better, recognizing the injustices against some CP families, and what prejudice and ignorance can do."

Taking a cue from Deanna and other young people in his program, O.D. (Bill) Cole is planning refinements for the next monitor course, to emphasize broader goals. Like the teenagers themselves, he sees it as much more than a super sitting service. "If, through our program," he says, "we can affect the lives of X number of young people so that they will enter worthwhile careers and become substantial citizens—this, to me, is the payoff."

1. Don't Call Them Baby Sitters, Golin M, *Saturday Evening Post,* Jun 20, 1959.

After Dynamite Downs an Airliner

Forty-three years after Theodore Roosevelt's savior waited beside an assassin in Milwaukee, two reporters on a busman's holiday mingled with a different crowd of onlookers in Denver to glimpse an accused multiple killer. Theirs turned out to be more than a mere glimpse.

Unable to find steady work to support his family, John Gilbert Graham had enough time on his hands on Nov 1, 1955 to help his mother pack her three suitcases. She would be flying on a United Air Lines flight to visit her sister in Genevieve MO. And she was worried. Mrs. Daisie King, who'd had two other husbands after Jack Graham was born, confided to him a premonition of doom.

After he noticed that hinges on the suitcase were breaking, he went to a neighborhood hardware store and bought a couple of sturdy straps to girdle the packed luggage. At Denver's Stapleton Field, Graham stopped at a vending machine and bought a $37,500 flight insurance policy on his mother's life. She signed it, naming her son as beneficiary.

Mrs. King embraced Jack and, with trepidation, boarded the DC-6B airliner. Eleven minutes after takeoff, the plane exploded over a farm in Longmont, Colo. All 44 aboard were killed.

Investigators determined that a dynamite bomb caused the blast. They checked airport flight insurance machines, found a record of Jack Graham's policy, and questioned him.[1]

In a pre-arraignment appearance Nov. 17, 1955 at the U.S. District Court in Denver, Graham heard federal prosecutors claim they had a "written admission" that he had packed dynamite in his mother's suitcase, allegedly to collect on her insurance. Following procedure in a federal criminal case, the U.S. Attorney told the court he would not elaborate on the evidence before the trial.[2]

By coincidence, I was among rubberneckers outside a fourth floor courtroom as federal marshals led Graham, handcuffed and shackled, to a van headed for the county jail. With me was Don Carter, news director for WMBI, a Chicago radio station affiliated with the Moody Bible Institute.

As we watched the prisoner being led into the van, a wild thought came to mind. In the spirit of a hyped up reporter on a busman's holiday, I asked Turner, "What say we try interviewing him? Nothing on our schedule tonight."

An hour earlier, we had arrived in Denver on a government transport plane with a dozen other Midwest reporters and editors as guests of the U.S. Air Force. We would be shown NORAD, the new Air Force electronic early-alert system at Boulder, CO. First, though, we decided to join the crowd inside the courthouse.

"Why not," Turner agreed. "What have we got to lose, except maybe a turn-down by the warden? Besides, here's a good way to try out my new wire recorder." It was a heavy contraption; antique today; smaller, light-weight tape recorders had not yet become widely available commercially.

Convincing the Denver jail warden turned out to be a snap. "Sure, come on over," he told Turner in a preliminary phone call. "I'm from Chicago and still listen to WMBI's programs."

A half-hour later in the office of warden Gordon Dolliver—he resembled a Hollywood mob figure from central casting—we waited for the inmate to be brought up and offered answers to questions as Dolliver reminisced about visits to Chicago: When will Wrigley Field start running night games? Will they ever bring the Criminal Courts building to the Loop? How is the new subway system working out?

Before long, in shuffled Jack Graham wearing orange prison garb and escorted by two armed guards. He was hobbled by clanking shackles and handcuffs. The impromptu recorded interview began with an effort toward leading up slowly to the allegations against him, and his responses.

Mainly because our knowledge of the case was so limited, based solely on a hasty reading of Denver's two leading newspapers during the taxi ride to the jail, early questions were poorly prepared, stilted, and banal:

Are they treating you all right? "Yeah, I guess so." Food OK? "Not bad." Anything we can get you—newspaper, magazine? "No." Would you like us to bring you a Bible [Turner asking]? "Well, if you want to. Sure."

Do you miss your family? No answer. Your friends? No answer.

Your mother? Again silence, as the prisoner surveyed the room, took in the surroundings—an unoccupied black leather couch, the high ceiling, the warden leaning back in an upholstered chair behind his bare desktop, dull gray walls, a clerk taking notes. He seemed uncomfortable near the introduced two reporters with their strange, humming machine between them. And, of course, the scowling guards pressing against him. The interview continued:

Do you understand the charges against you? "Yes."

Have you seen an attorney? "A lawyer is coming tomorrow."
Were you especially close to your mother? "Yeah."
Did you attend her funeral? "Yes."
How long did you stay? "As long as I could."
Did you go with the rest of your family? With your sister? "That's right."
Is she praying for you? "I haven't seen her."
Do you feel we're questioning you fairly? "Don't make any difference to me."
Is there anything you'd like to say on your own behalf on this whole situation? "No."
About anything? "No."
Anything we can do for you, besides bring the Bible? "No. Everything is just fine."
You realize you're going to be brought to trial, don't you? "Yeah."
And there's a possibility you'll be convicted? "That's right."
And the sort of punishment for a crime of this type? "That's right."
How would you feel about meeting your Creator if that happens? "You gotta go sometime."
What have you done to prepare yourself? "I didn't know you had to do anything."
Mr. Graham, what made you confess?[3]

Now came a loud burst of response. The prisoner shot up from his chair, his shackles rattling. "I didn't do it," he shouted. "There is no real confession. They beat it out of me. Said they'd arrest my wife and take our two kids.

One by one, jaws dropped and there was a collective gasp. First the warden's jaw, next the two guards', then the trembling jaw of a woman clerk. As wire in the recording spool kept unwinding, the guards hustled Graham out of the warden's side door and headed back to his cell. Nobody uttered a word until Carter and I slipped away lugging the 12-pound recording machine. As one, we muttered, "Thanks, warden."

What now? We discussed whether this was a story for our Chicago editors. "It doesn't fit my broadcast news format," said Turner.

"Nor mine at City News Bureau," I concluded. "Yet, it *is* a big story. CNB is owned by the Chicago newspapers, but why would their editors care about a Denver police case or any other non-local event?"

In fact, a momentous non-local event did originate from City News Bureau 14 years earlier. On a relatively news-quiet Sunday in 1941, a reporter at the Damon Avenue police station on the city's near-northwest side was slowly twisting a dial on the desk sergeant's short-wave radio when they heard the static-punctuated voice of an amateur radio operator telling another "ham" that "bombs are falling all over Honolulu."

The eavesdropping reporter could hear explosions in the background of the radio transmission. He phoned what he had heard to his city editor, who immediately sent bulletins to the CNB's four main newspapers and the member Associated Press. It caught the AP by surprise and within seconds the report was on news wires worldwide. Thus City News Bureau was first to break the news of Japan's attack on Pearl Harbor.[4]

We decided to offer the story free to a local news outlet. After a *Denver Post* editor demurred, I phoned the *Rocky Mountain News* city desk, saying: "Graham has recanted. We just finished interviewing him at the jail. We have a recording in which he denies confessing."

Within minutes, a reporter arrived at our hotel room and took notes from the recording. In next morning's edition, the story was on the streets with photos from the court appearance occupying the front page under a banner headline, "DYNAMITER CHANGES HIS STORY." [2] The *News* had scooped the *Post*, and the story landed on the Associated Press national wire.

The news created an uproar in the federal prosecutor's office. The public defender who had been appointed to represent Graham arrived at the jail early to begin replanning a strategy for his case. Arresting officers and prosecutors wondered what went wrong with what they felt was solid evidence.

While the scooped *Denver Post* hastened to recover, the *Rocky Mountain News* was nimbler,[2] sending its star police reporter first to warden Dolliver for a more thorough interview with Graham. At that point, the clamor from reporters for the *Denver Post* and Associated Press became so intense that warden Dolliver set up a wide-open news conference at the jail. Graham continued to proclaim his innocence.

In later editions, the *News* became heady about its double-whammy "scoop," crowing, "This [is a] first interview"[5]—failing to mention that Carter and I had handed the initial interview to the *News*. Here was a curious bent in news competition.

Still in our hotel room, Carter and I charted new directions for the story. At convention headquarters of the Radio and Television News Directors Association, which recently had accepted me as a member, I suggested to the program chairman that playing the recording might put a current-events twist on their afternoon session. He agreed and the event earned an RTNDA item[4] and a story in next day's news.[6]

But before the meeting began, I headed for a bookstore to keep a promise. I bought a Bible for Jack Graham and delivered it to the jail's reception gate.

Wait. There's more, a third story angle by two nervy newsmen.

Remembering that former President Dwight Eisenhower's widow Mamie lived in Denver, I tracked down the phone number of her pastor. Our conversation:

Q—Have you heard about Jack Graham's claim of innocence in the airliner bombing? A—Yes, the story just came over on the TV news.

Q—Have you considered counseling him? A—As a matter of fact, I was planning to head out for the jail this afternoon.

When the pastor did visit Graham, that made another scoop for the *Post* over the *News.*

How many other news stories, Turner and I ask each other, are born and thrive this way? Further, was it wrong, even illegal, to intrude on a government institution and its warden, circumventing official and judicial channels, in gaining access to a prosecutorial subject—for the purpose of obtaining a news story? And where was the justification for pursuing a story without editorial assignment or supervision?

I refer these and related questions to academic journalists, ethicists, and privacy proponents. But for that time and in that place, Turner and I stumbled upon a major story, developed it, and followed through with reporter-initiated features, simply because we believed that news people go where the news is, even if they help it along. Throughout our unusual quest, there was no monetary or other personal gain. So, we concluded, nobody was harmed.

On return to Chicago, having socialized with other RTNDA members and also fulfilled the second part of the original flight plan—touring the Air Force global defense alert facility, I read that Graham had repudiated his recantation and was convicted because of damning testimony. Prosecutors for the first time had revealed crucial details to the court: Investigators at the crash scene found an alarm clock linked to a battery-operated timer.

Shrewd detective work established that Graham had been identified by a hardware store clerk, from whom he bought the reinforcing straps for his mother's suitcase, as the man who also purchased the alarm clock and the timing mechanism. Confronted with complete evidence, Graham admitted that he had packed 23 sticks of dynamite with its lethal trigger in the luggage. He changed his plea to guilty and threw himself at the mercy of the court.

U. S. District Judge James M. Neland offered no mercy. A few weeks later, John Gilbert Graham, age 23, was executed in Colorado's gas chamber.[5]

Later I learned that the journalistic venture, even though it resulted in Graham's true guilt, had gone unnoticed by City News Bureau editors: "You did what? Interviewed a multiple killer in jail and got a front-page exclusive? Oh, come on!" *Chicago Tribune* past issues revealed that the newspaper indeed had run the early AP story, naming Carter and me as the jailhouse interviewers.[6]

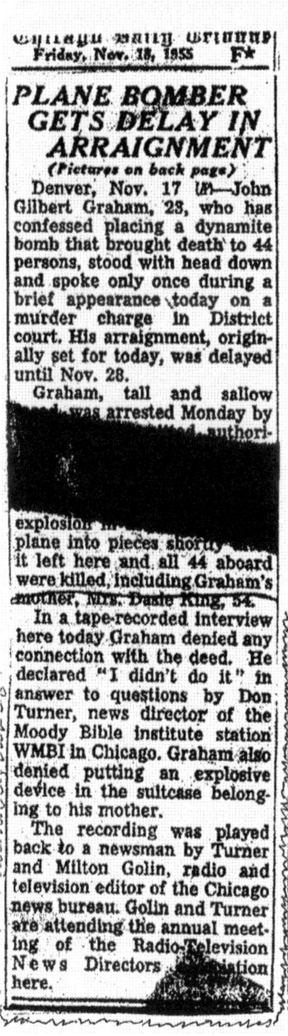

Friday, Nov. 18, 1955 F★

PLANE BOMBER GETS DELAY IN ARRAIGNMENT

(Pictures on back page)

Denver, Nov. 17 (AP)—John Gilbert Graham, 23, who has confessed placing a dynamite bomb that brought death to 44 persons, stood with head down and spoke only once during a brief appearance today on a murder charge in District court. His arraignment, originally set for today, was delayed until Nov. 28.

Graham, tall and sallow [illegible] was arrested Monday by [illegible] authori- [illegible] explosion [illegible] plane into pieces shortly [illegible] it left here and all 44 aboard were killed, including Graham's mother, Mrs. Dasie King, 54.

In a tape-recorded interview here today Graham denied any connection with the deed. He declared "I didn't do it" in answer to questions by Don Turner, news director of the Moody Bible Institute station WMBI in Chicago. Graham also denied putting an explosive device in the suitcase belonging to his mother.

The recording was played back to a newsman by Turner and Milton Golin, radio and television editor of the Chicago news bureau. Golin and Turner are attending the annual meeting of the Radio-Television News Directors [illegible] here.

However, one City News milestone was reached. General manager Isaac Gershman determined it was the first time in the Bureau's 65-year history that a Bible had been approved on an expense account.

1. Dynamiter Denies Story, Nakulla A, *Rocky Mountain News,* Nov 18, 1955.

2. Guilt Denied in Plane Bombing, *New York Times,* Nov 19, 1955.

3. Plane Bomber Gets Delay, (AP) *Chicago Tribune,* Nov 18, 1955.

4. Behind the Front Page, Dornfeld AA, Academy Chicago Publishers 1983.

5. ibid *Rocky Mountain News.*

6. Turner and Golin Take Bus Driver's Holiday, *RTNDA Newsletter,* Jan 1956...Illinois .News Broadcasters Association Newsletter, Jan 1956.

7. Letter to John Temple, editor and publisher of *Rocky Mountain News,*

How Computer Therapy Helps Autistic Children

Like cerebral palsy youngsters who are helped by medically trained teenage monitors, therapy for autistic children involves its own high drama. Unusual health benefits via computers and the Internet illustrate life-uplifting experiences.

It's a true celebration for the 14-year-old youth. For years he had suffered in silence and dread whenever other students approached with a friendly greeting. Autism prevented clear response. Now he is chattering away on a World Wide Web forum,. "Long live the Internet," He exults in an online discussion. "People can see the real me, not just how I react superficially or not at all with other people."

During another Internet "chat" session, a young housewife explains why she prefers online to face-to-face interaction: "Ordinarily, the giving of support involves being with someone. That's always draining to me. If someone does give support in person, I'll have to spend some time recovering from the experience."

Mae, a 12-year-old eighth grader from Long Island, NY, stands before a national autistic society conference to describe a similar feeling. Then she tells how getting a notebook computer changed all that: "It allows me to do my work as quickly as the other students...One girl was always teasing me because I was autistic. Now I know how to ignore it."

Those experiences are not exceptional in cyberspace. While cerebral palsy youngsters in Phoenix, AZ are helped by trained young monitors, other afflicted children across the country find therapy in computer use.

Along the dozens of electronic highways devoted to autism—with their many Web site stops for forums, chats, interview sessions, research probings, and morale boosters, a little-noticed yet immense revolution is taking place. The computer is seen as a haven, a social catalyst, and a therapeutic key for autistic people.

The phenomenon is being compared to the beneficial effects for the blind when Braille was introduced, and for the deaf when sign language was developed.

The revolution continues as, day by day, more autistics visit Internet sites designed to meet their wants and needs. In fact, some of them have set up and run the sites, with autistic participants in mind.

"There is no reason why this growth should not continue at a great pace," says Temple Grandin, PhD, an authority in the field and herself autistic.[13x] "Here is a condition twice as common as blindness. It can be just as disabling or more so." In an August 1997 interview with me for the newsmagazine *Computers & Medicine,*[1] she pointed out that an autistic person's typical problems with eye contact and body language of other people don't occur in computer use, adding:

"How the computer works is how my mind works. When I try to think and figure out, it is like searching on the 'Net. The way Web pages are linked is associative, not linear. I used to believe that's how everybody thinks.

"Today many people with autism are fascinated with computers and become very good at programming. Problems that they have with eye contact and awkward gestures are not visible on the Internet, and typewritten messages avoid many of the social problems of face-to-face contact. The Internet may be the best thing for improving an autistic person's social life."[2]

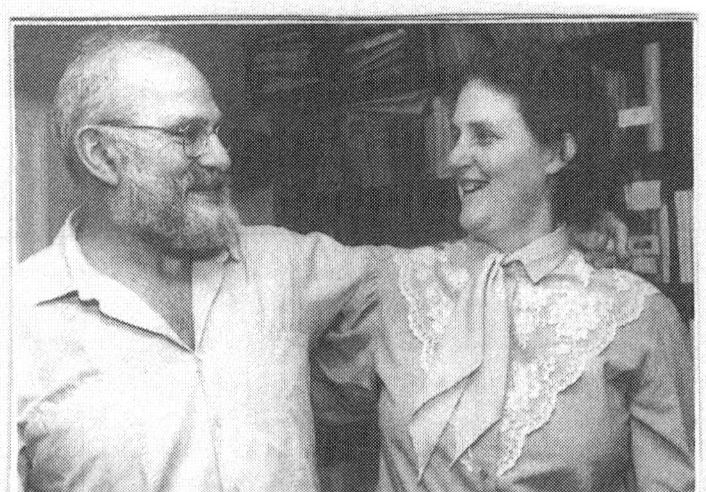

Autism expert Temple Grandin (right) with author/neurologist Oliver Sacks. M.D. She writes that "the Internet may be the best thing for improving an autistic person's life."
Photo copyright Rosalie Winard, courtesy Computers & Medicine.

Grandin's words underscore her expertise, as told in her memoir, "Thinking in Pictures and Other Reports from My life With Autism." Her experiences are reminiscent of electrical wizard and inventor Nikola Tesla, whose innovations helped generate today's computer world. Shortly before he died in 1943, Tesla wrote how he would visualize entire new circuits in great detail—and then easily make all connections on a board.

That is an autistic trait, sharing comparable status with Microsoft chief Bill Gates. He rocks during business meetings and while flying on airplanes; autistic children and other adults also rock back and forth. But is autism a correct diagnosis simply because of an isolated trait or traits?

How many people can be classified as autistic in the U.S.? About 800,000, based on an incidence of 1.5 per 100,000, according to the Autism Society of America, headquartered in Bethesda, MD. Only 20% of this number can be regarded as highly functional enough to operate a computer, Grandin estimates, and perhaps 10% of those—or 16,000—currently visit Internet sites.

About half of all autistics are nonverbal. Therefore, it would be grossly overoptimistic to conclude that the many and varied gains for autistic people that can be attributable to computer use are widespread—at least for now. Of course any advancement can represent a highly laudable trend. Over a period of 10 weeks, as editor of *Computers & Medicine,* I visited 11 autism-related Web sites plus 37 of their links, to get a feel for the varied activities and commentary. Here is a sampling of what I learned:

- Interview comments of neurologist Oliver Sacks, MD, author of such best-sellers as *Awakenings, an Anthropologist on Mars,* and *The Man who Mistook His Wife for a Hat.* [Excerpt: Q—"Do you have a neurological disorder that compels you to examine neurological disorders?" A—"I feel distracted much of the time, darting from one thing to another, but I think there is some sort of consistency or tenacity to it."]
- Another interview, this one of Temple Grandin and conducted by author Harvey Blume. [Excerpt:

  Q—"Why do you often use the analogy of wiring to describe autistic thought processes?" A—"I use the Internet talk because there is nothing out there closer to how I think."] Because many autistics are skilled computer programmers, says Blume, "they look at the protocols governing exchange between networked machines as models for the sort of structured interchange they are most comfortable with."]
- On the Living Forum e-mail page, an autistic man expresses his condition: "Imagine you a are surrounded by 10 people rapidly talking to you at the same time (a politician answering questions, for instance), and this would go on for several hours. You would want to run into a small room

and lock the door behind you. This is how I feel when I'm talking to two people—or one person sometimes. E-mail is best for me."

- An "Autism Checklist" illustrates 18 typical symptoms such as echolalia (repeating words or phrases in place of normal language), inappropriate laughing or giggling, no real fear of dangers, and tantrums. Researchers also report ultrasensitivity to sharp noises and intense desire not to socialize face-to-face. This might explain why many amateur ("ham") radio operators, because of their autism, prefer to communicate via Morse Code. Phonic communications would require interpreting voice intonations.

A speech by a 12-year-old girl in which she calls being "literal" a serious problem: "My teacher said we should be quiet, not even breathe. I thought he was trying to kill us."

I found an index of 962 worldwide Internet addresses of pages and links on autism and related neurological disorders. These sites include newsgroups, treatment plans, research. in progress, diagnostic standards, likely causes of autism, book recommendations for parents and siblings, support resources, social and educational implications and strategies, individual schooling programs, conferences, social studies, rehabilitation computer games, poetry by autistics, and family stories.

There are also Web sites designed to help autistic adults dress appropriately for job-search. Hobbies are described and there are detailed responses to a recurrent question: "How can I relate to neurologically typical people?"—NTs in the autism community's parlance.

Sexuality is another topic. Describing his thinking-in-pictures mentality, a 26-year-old computer professional tells an Independent Living session on the Internet that as a teenager he imagined orgasm as "a burst-mode file transfer over a high-bandwidth circuit."

Merely because many autistic people wish to relate to NTs does not necessarily mean they want to be neurologically typical. Grandin, for one, treasures her ability to think in pictures and says she would not trade that faculty for a culture based primarily on emotion. Studies of deaf communities indicate a comparable goal, as seen in continuing debate over sign language vs. lip reading for predominant education.

To cynics who would argue that computer-using autistics represent only a small fraction of all those (800,000) with this disorder, several questions pose rebuttal:

—Who can predict what major therapeutic gains will ensue for the estimated 400,000 relatively uncommunicative autistics—as their more articulating counterparts on the Internet interact with one another and with medical and social scientists?

—Who could have foreseen that the advents of Braille, sign language, and cochlear implants would create the broad-based "revolutions" that have benefited much larger numbers of the blind and deaf than was first thought?

—Who can reasonably question that the prospect of finding a therapeutic key to unlock yet-undiscovered treatments for more of those seemingly intractable autistics is considerably enhanced by advances in electronic communications?

Meanwhile, a truer image is being defined and refined in the new world opening for autistics on the Internet. It is beginning to supplant the long-held stereotype of a person who keeps rocking back and forth, is averse to touch, shuns self-care, cannot connect with other people, and whose sole skill is to instantaneously multiply large numbers in his head like the character portrayed by Dustin Hoffman in the movie "Rain Man."

Anyone who visits autism sites on the Internet will see a multi-layered different side of the human subject. There, they will find many autistic youngsters doing the very thing that the syndrome is supposed to prevent them from doing. They are interacting with others and defying their "communication disorder" label—in the process celebrating the electronic medium that enables them to do so.

1. Autism: The Internet As Haven, Educator, Social Catalyst & Therapeutic Key, Golin M, *Computers & Medicine,* Aug 1997.

Dr. Von Braun Plans a Mars Rescue

Forty years before autism yielded new vistas of Internet therapy for untreated kids, more primitive computer systems were exploring a space-age medical frontier. The quest for "health in the heavens"[1] moved forward years before the rocket launch of the first man into orbit, Yuri Gegarin of the USSR.

Wernher von Braun was certain that his plan to reach an astronaut on Mars would work. But would the vital next step succeed: rescuing and bringing the man back to safety if his exploratory mission had stranded him on the remote planet?

Fellow PhD aerospace physicist Fred Singer was skeptical. While on a barge inching along the San Antonio River one November day in 1958—how ironic for men whose ideas were driven by superspeed travel—they hashed out the plusses and minuses of the hypothetical rescue:

Is the dropping of an added oxygen supply an urgent first goal? Should the recovery vehicle land on Mars, or would it be more feasible to retrieve the survivor via a pickup system aloft—to the Mars-orbiting mother ship? If pickup is decided, how would a lifeline be sent down—by helical descent or a more pinpointed method? Precision won out in the discussion.

Singer computed a trajectory that would sweep up the astronaut. Von Braun figured out how to adjust the velocity of the rescue vehicle by factoring in Mars gravity with centripetal and cetrifugal forces in the sweep.

So animated was the give and take of von Braun and Singer that a dozen other scientists on the barge huddled around them in awe to catch every word. All the passengers were on break between sessions of an international conference on the physics and medicine of outer space. As an assistant editor preparing a paper for *The Journal of the American Medical Association,* I was also among the eavesdroppers.

"Sure," said Singer, "like you say, shoot a line from the mother ship to precisely boomerang for plucking the astronaut's grounded space capsule. But won't the tremendous centripetal returning force snap off his head?"

"I'm working on that problem," von Braun countered.

For nearly two hours, as the barge passed through San Antonio's business district and under bridges connecting sidewalks 20 feet above the river, the men's dialogue parried one another's ideas on the theoretically deadly event millions of miles from Earth. They never did complete the "rescue," not during the river journey anyway.

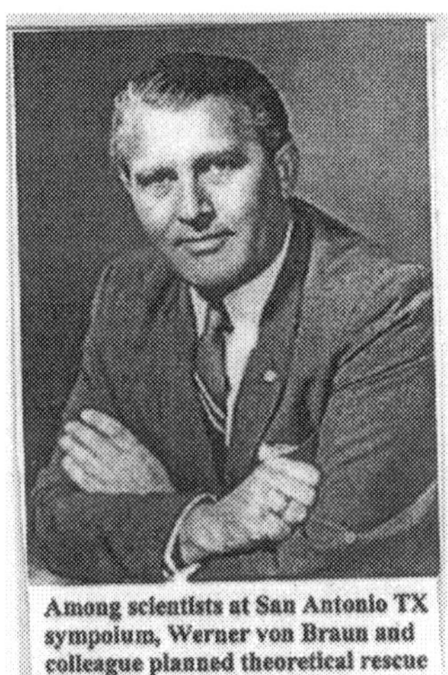

Among scientists at San Antonio TX sympoium, Werner von Braun and colleague planned theoretical rescue of astronaut stranded onMars.

Back at the Hilton Hotel conference center, barge passengers rejoined more than 700 other astrophysicists, aerospace engineers and scientists, and aviation medicine specialists in lectures, seminars, and panel discussions. Singer joined a panel on speed-of-light, problems of rescue in space, and closed ecologic systems.

Von Braun's lecture described his proposed orbiting space station and drew on his pioneering V-2 rocket for Hitler in World War II. He and his team of 126 rocket specialists at Peenemunde later surrendered to American forces in order to achieve more notable successes in space science and engineering. Von Braun became a U.S. citizen in 1955.

University of Iowa physicist James A.Van Allen told a seminar that "the moon is old hat," adding: "We would like to emphasize interplanetary or space probes rather than merely moon shots. We are concentrating now on probing Mars and Venus."

But what about space-age medical problems? How close are they to solution? Citing an ironic time warp, Van Allen recalled a historic event, noting that the same questions had been posed five generations earlier: In 1785, French scientists sent a hen, a duck, and a goat up in a balloon 8,000 feet across the English Channel to test "animal durability at great heights." When only the hen appeared worse for wear on landing, said Van Allen, they deduced that space flight was bad for chickens—until somebody found feathers in the goat's mouth.

At the San Antonio conference, medical scientists were exerting a more upward-look-with-feet-on ground. Some were probing survival needs at an altitude where blood effervesces. Others were testing muscular coordination, vision, and blood pressure in a gravity-free state. Still other doctors were puzzling over delusions that cobweb human consciousness under the stress of relentless concentration on instrument panels.

These physicians were not romping recklessly in the wispy world of science fiction, making playful studies of such fantasies as antigravity belts and disintegrator pistols. Theirs was an earthly, practical assault on space medicine problems of the immediate future.

One seminar conclusion was that "everything about the effect of space flight on the human body has a distinct value to generations of people who spend the rest of their lives on solid earth. This new knowledge may answer such questions as:

How can the harmful effects of ozone, occurring at the fringe of outer space as well as in manufacturing operations, be countered more efficiently? Why can greater understanding of cosmic rays hundreds of miles above the earth contribute to radiobiology? What will the orthopedist and neurologist learn about reflexes in the gravity-free state? How can the internist benefit from the knowledge of organic functioning during prolonged periods of weightlessness among astronauts who spend dayless and nightless time in an inky void that is pierced by a searchlight sun and the bluish glow of once-secure earth?

Beyond the questions there is recognition that every problem in space medicine touches upon some nonmedical field: psychology, astrophysics, biochemistry, engineering, biology. Equally tough are problems of aerodynamic heating, diet, communication, equilibrium, and breathing. And as some problems are scratched off as solved, others loom into view:[2]

Can humans ever adapt naturally to higher and higher altitudes on earth? When will we be able to safely stop a pilot from spinning as rapidly as 200 rpm as he escapes from a disabled plane at very high altitude?

What can be done to counteract "empty field myopia," the nearsightedness that is expected to attack even normal eyes in space, where there is no reference focus point? How can we reduce the physiologic damage caused by a rocket ship's intense noise during takeoff—and solve the psychological problem of extended deathly silence afterward?

All of this continuing search for knowledge could one day help rescue an astronaut marooned on an a different planet—via a refined method that was only theorized by Wernher von Braun and Fred Singer aboard a San Antonio river barge in 1958. Their effort did not quite succeed then, opening the way for future scientists to solve these problems.

If anything on planet Earth can be as inhospitable to humans as Mars, one need only experience the storm-ridden region of the Himalayan mountain range that separates Burma, India, and China—known as The Hump. In World War II, American fighting forces there faced deadly encounters as daunting as those confronting today's astronauts.

1. Health in the Heavens, Golin M, *JAMA,* Jun 15, 1957.

2. ibid.

3. The Moon Is Old Hat, Golin, M, *JAMA,* Jan 31, 1959.

Danger and Diversion in the Shadow of Mount Everest

"...In the winter it gets so cold that the wings of some planes ice up, making them lose altitude. In blizzard conditions, with winds of up to 200 miles an hour, often visibility is impossible. Pilots remember flying across the Himalayas and never seeing anything until five minutes before landing. When it isn't freezing or snowing, the monsoons swamp everything. Rainfall can be 15 inches a day in the wet season..."

So here is the hotshot Army Air Corps navigator in 1945, his logbook of 14 global ferrying missions[1] still crammed into a back pocket of his jungle shorts. He stares in puzzlement at his Jeep's trailer, stuck in the ditch.

All because of a roadside navigation error. How mortifying! Onlooking soldiers gawk, and snicker at the gleaming navigator wings on his shirt. Nobody had explained why, when backing a trailer, you rotate the steering wheel opposite the usual turning direction.

This is no ordinary road. It is the Burma Road, arguably World War II's most strategic line of communication and supply, a marvel of repetitious hairpin-curve construction winding across the Himalayas.

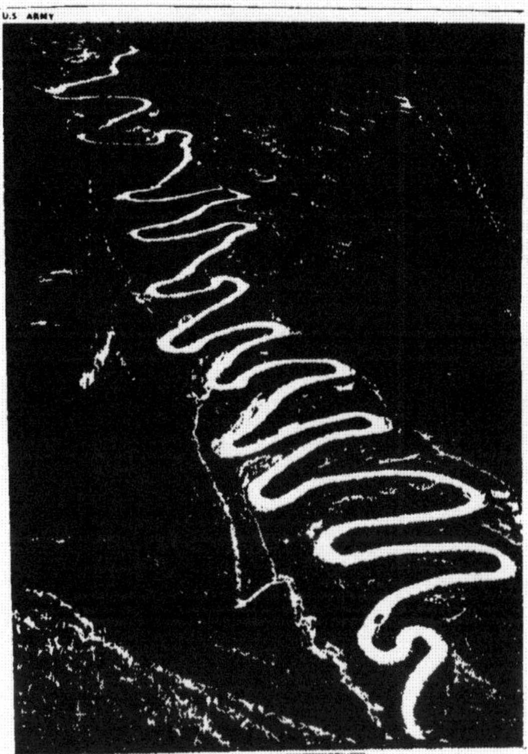

View of Burma Road, showing series of 21 famous steps of hairpin turns on Himalayan "Hump."

It is the most important land route to China for carrying armament and both American and Chinese troops against the Japanese enemy.

Still connected to the ditched trailer, the Jeep sprawls askew the Burma Road, blocking lanes of vital traffic. For an hour, truckers blast their air horns. Drivers of Jeeps, troop carriers, and other vehicles honk in multi-tones. Some also curse. It isn't easy to unhitch the trailer so that the Jeep can clear the lanes.

The errant navigator had not watched closely while the motor pool guys did the hookup. So how can he unhook? He tries loosening a bolt here, bending a latch there, kicking at the damn joint. Nothing works.

Finally, a tanker truck driver, a corporal who has done most of the yelling, ambles over and separates the two vehicles and curbs the Jeep. Traffic moves.

But a problem remains: how to raise the freed trailer to road level without losing its heavy—and precious—load of sand. Precious, because it is a key ingredient of concrete floors that the navigator and other air base personnel are rushing to build for their thatched-roof "bashas," living quarters.

It turns out that shoveling of sand is unnecessary. Somebody has reached the motor pool and soon a crew with block and tackle is hauling the trailer out of the ditch. The navigator again heads for the basha-building site.

The urgent construction knows no rank. Corporals and captains dig foundations in the parched soil. Majors and privates erect sturdy bamboo poles and rolls of screening for roof supports and sidewalls. Lieutenants and sergeants churn the sand with water and bags of cement. In three or four days, weather forecasters tell them, the seemingly ceaseless monsoon rains will begin.

Facing the base commander will not be easy. The colonel has heard loudly from a half-dozen equal- or higher-ranking officers stalled on the Road. He's eager to dress down the one at fault. The navigator knows it will be useless to explain. But he never has to.

By the time he arrives at base headquarters, the commander has cooled down, still distraught from news that still another C-46 tanker plane has crashed after its pilot loses his way crossing the Hump to China. Records show that the pilot has defied regulations by failing to attend a required navigation and weather briefing before takeoff.

The colonel sends word to his adjutant, "Tell that briefing navigator to return to duty. We'll get back to him later." A form letter reprimand follows, but in the hubbub over the plane crash, it does not appear in the navigator's file. Paperwork is in a shambles.

When a monsoon season approaches, such a lapse in record-keeping is not unusual at the Myitkyina (pronounced MISH-in-aw) air base. In the frantic atmosphere of move it move it move it before the long rains, schedules compress.

The mess hall is full two hours before the regular breakfast time. Basha construction crews are hammering and sawing and pouring concrete mix at deadline pace. The twin engines of the C-46 cargo and aircraft fuel tanker planes are revving up on tarmacs in groups of three and four, instead of singly, to accelerate the sequence of take-offs.

Then the skies open and time slows. Flights continue but at a reduced pace, and ground maintenance crews resume inventory tasks. Squads of motor pool noncoms sweep up the debris of hasty repair work. Many pilots, aircraft engineers, radio operators, and other crew members put finishing touches on their bashas, relieved to be out of their makeshift tents at this 1304th Army Air Forces Battalion Unit.

"How about a beer?" Red, the former Chicago police reporter turned navigator, calls out to his basha mates the evening of the first downpour. "Sure." two pilots yell back. He heads for the corner below-concrete storage bin and reaches down. There, staring at him, are the piercing eyes of a cobra, sharing the cool space with cans of Budweiser. "Forget it," a shaken Red hastily tells the others. All agree to let the cobra stay put until there is a safe retrieval strategy.

To a steady degree, certain stress levels drop as the rainwater rises. The three weather and navigational briefing officers now enjoy a respite from full duty as fewer Hump flights take off and land. There's time for occasional cribbage and pinochle, even blackjack.

But at another level, the stress of boredom amid continuing plane crashes (averaging three or four per week) takes its toll. At the end of World War II, 4,000 U.S. air crew members will have died in Hump trips.

Drinking increases at the air base. The three navigators turned card players begin sniping at one another. Tidbits in letters from home, shared earlier in an atmosphere of warmth and smiles, become fodder for slurs and ridicule.

Joe Shomo from Pittsburgh becomes the butt of gibes about his coming civilian career as a dentist. Red snorts his views: "You play that nine like you put in a filling, and I'm out of your dental chair pronto. Gad, what grubby fingers you got there, Doc."

Bill Graham is targeted for being namby-pamby about his lack of focus on planned college courses: "Sure you want to play that card, Bill? Can't you make up your mind about *anything?* God, what a loser!"

They in turn ride Red about letters from his loved one, a married mother of two: "Hey, instant Daddyo, what does her husband say about you two? You can sure pick your women, like the lousy cards you deal."

Today, in retrospect, it is apparent that unjustified feelings of guilt were a factor in turning enjoyable card games into arenas of discord. One rationale might be denial: *We* can't be blamed for the fiery smashup at the end of the runway. *We* didn't overload the C-46 tanker.

The day-to-day seeming lightness of activity masks the dead seriousness of operations at Myityina Airfield. For here is much more than a mere wayside point on the Burma Road, more than just a jumping off place for China destinations. It is a hard-fought strategic junction.

Myitkyina marked the final victorious thrust of Merrill's Marauders, a group of American irregulars under Col. Frank Merrill. In five major and 30 minor engagements, though vastly outnumbered, they defeated veteran soldiers of the Japanese 18th division. Climaxing their behind-the-lines operations with the capture of Myitkyina Airfield, they gained the only all-weather air base in northern Burma.

In the little-publicized China-Burma-India (CBI) theater of war, tens of thousands of Allied soldiers tied down a million-man Japanese force in China—a force that would have otherwise confronted General Douglas MacArthur's Pacific island-hopping campaign.[2] Twin-engine transport planes that fly the Hump from Myitkyina in all kinds of weather, day and night, cannot rise above 27,500 feet. In some places the mountains that these aircraft cross in zig zag fashion are higher. Mount Everest, the planet's highest point, peaks at 29,028 feet. So planes must zig zag along valleys below lower peaks.

Adding to the peril is the weather. In winter it gets so cold that the wings of some planes ice up, making them lose altitude and crash. During blizzard conditions, with winds up to 200 miles an hour, visibility is impossible—zero.[3] When it isn't freezing and snowing, the monsoons swamp everything. Rainfall is 15 inches a day at the height of the wet season. Pilots remember flying across the Himalayas and never seeing anything until 15 minutes before landing.[4]

When crew members fly across the Hump, each is issued a vest that has 36 pockets. These contain emergency rations, maps of the area printed on silk, jungle knife and saw, and other items that might help survival in a jungle.

A Chinese flag is sewn inside the flight jacket with a message in four dialects. It reads: We are friends trying to help defeat a common enemy. The two top buttons of the survival vest can be removed. By placing the magnetized one atop the other, these make a crude but effective compass.

Even today, the U.S. Air Force will not reveal how many planes did not complete the 500-mile flight across the Hump—crashing on takeoff or landing, getting lost in transit, shot down by Japanese fighter squadrons. "Roughly five hundred" is the figure cited unofficially in briefing sessions.

That number is considered accurate by the late Wilbur G. Davidson of Stowe, Ohio, who kept a detailed diary while serving as a civilian rubber engineer for the B. F. Goodrich Company in the CBI theater. He and other aeronautical experts had been assigned there to reduce casualties by developing, installing, and maintaining anti-icing equipment on aircraft.

Davidson writes in his diary: "I had access to a lot of confidential information on aircraft losses. During the time we were there, between 500 and 600 planes were lost flying the Hump—some to enemy action, some to weather, some to pilot error."[5]

At an April, 2000 reunion of 300 CBI veterans in Kunming, China one pilot, Robert Friedman of Port Charlotte, FL, recalled Hump flight conditions before there were briefing-meteorology officers at Myitkyina: "In those days, they'd hand you your orders and tell you, 'Find your own way across the Hump.' Later, they established flight routes."

That was the chief problem for early Hump flyers. They had to find a route north of the then-Japanese air base at Myitkyina. But the farther north they flew, the higher the Himalayas got—and the more daunting the trip became.

The main product transported was aircraft gasoline, planes filled with 55-gallon barrels of it for Allied forces in China. The need for fuel was desperate because the Japanese were blockading the China coast.

For the three briefing officers at Myitkyina, fantasies paint scenarios involving the conscientious, hard-working Red Cross nurses on the base—how they supposedly spend their days and nights. Scenarios include singalongs with bawdy verses like, "I'm Dreaming of a White Mistress."

There are moments of relaxing diversion: haggling with Burmese locals who peddle star sapphires, moonstones, rubies, and cat's eye gems...Night-time deer hunting from a Jeep...A hike in the jungle, punctuated by guffaws when Red stops to rest on what looks like a log.

The wakened 16-foot, wide-bodied giant python stirs, glances at the quick-rising sitter, then goes back to sleep. "Lot more exciting than steering that trailer into a ditch," mocks Joe Shomo. Still trembling, Red sulks.

One night at the officers' club, a pilot methodically feeds liquor to his pet rhesus monkey. Why is he enjoying the animal's drunken antics? Punishment, he replies.

Back from a Hump trip that afternoon, the pilot sees that the monkey has found two cartons of cigarettes in his foot locker, tearing up the cartons, unwrapping each pack, and neatly breaking each cigarette in two. The 800 butts are strewn around every bed, desk, and chair in the four-man basha.

The three briefing officers grasp opportunities to escape the monsoon briefly. They take turns hitching a plane ride to Calcutta for shrimp dinners at Dum Dum air base. They launch one-day mapping and compass-calibration missions to Ceylon, New Delhi, Singapore, and Shanghai (where they're told that the briefing officer moonlights as a downtown brothel operator.)

They sign on for humanitarian flights to Rangoon, air-dropping food, supplies, and medicines for a leper colony. And they fly the Hump to check out first-hand the best dog-leg routings along valleys, as well as around and between sub-Everest peaks.[6]

In addition, the briefing officers gauge levels of cloud cover and other weather conditions, to more accurately prepare pilots of succeeding flights. Good luck; weather can change every hour.

Another motivation for these flights across the Himalayas is breakfast at China destinations—Yunanni and Kunming, headquarters of the U. S. 14th Army Air Corps. There the fare is fresh eggs, welcome relief from the powdered eggs at Myitkyina.

Tales of what happens before, during, and after some of the journeys—whether true or false—become folklore. Pilots and ground maintenance crews tell of superstitious Chinese soldiers rushing close by whirling propellers in order to kill the accompanying "devil."

Trying to determine why they must trim the level of their C-47 plane frequently, a signal of reduced load (or so the story goes), the pilot and copilot peer back toward their load of Chinese soldiers. The passengers are playing a finger-showing game called "scissors." Losers are tossed out the open hatch.

In a reported practical joke on another transport of Chinese troops, the pilot and copilot rig coat hangers into the fingers of their service gloves and attach the handless and armless gloves to each of the plane's two operating controls. Switching to automatic pilot, they then scrunch out of view in opposing corners of the cockpit and gently push ajar the center doors. Within seconds, they hear anticipated screams from the soldiers, who are convinced that ghosts and/or devils have taken over the flight.

The briefing officers have their own favorite bit of folklore. But to them, as navigators, it rings true, not as a mere tale. One version has a second-lieutenant navigator placing his service pistol to the head of the captain pilot, risking court martial in order to force a change of course.

The twin-engine bomber is supposed to head east from Natal, Brazil for a fueling stop at Ascension Island in the South Atlantic, before continuing northeast to coastal Central Africa. But the pilot insists on flying directly to the African air base, 972 nautical miles farther. His route is certain to end in a crash at sea when the plane runs out of fuel.

When and where has this happened? What kind of bomber? Does it crash? Does the pilot change course? Then what? Where do you hear this story? Answers vary.

"I hear about it from the briefing officer at Ascension, who swears it's true," says Joe Shomo. "It is a B-25 bomber from Belem, Brazil, not Natal, in 1943. The pilot is a first lieutenant, not a captain, and he does change course. The navigator comes up for court martial but is not prosecuted. ATC officers in Tunis and Cairo tell me the same story."

Bill Graham says he hears the story from an Air Corps major in Khartoum, Egypt, adding, "You have it wrong. The plane is a B-26 bomber from somewhere else in Brazil, and it happens in 1944. The pilot changes course only after he and the copilot wrestle the gun away from the navigator. The way I hear it, the pilot and navigator are only reprimanded, for maybe court martial later."

Red, the journalist navigator from Chicago, tells Shomo and Graham that he's heard variations of the story at more than a half-dozen air bases and believes that elements of it are probably true. He says no more because his court martial is still possible.

Completion of military service in 1946, however, is without prosecution or even revelation of the mutiny. It remains secret for another 46 years. Now civilian news coverage, with its own high drama, resumes.

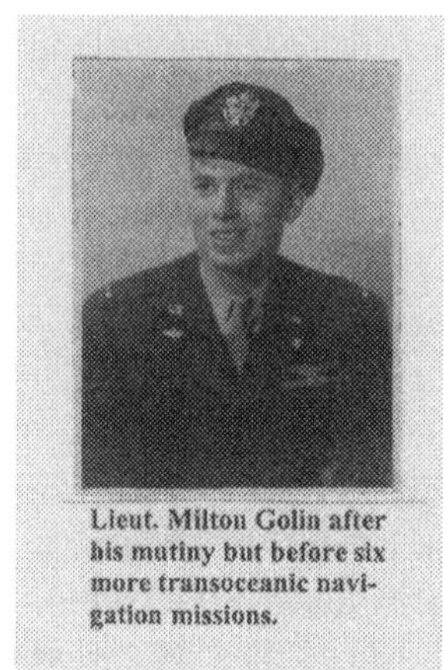

Lieut. Milton Golin after his mutiny but before six more transoceanic navigation missions.

1. Air Navigator's log book.
2. Self-published diary of W. Davidson 1978.
3. ibid. Hump Pilots Association newsletter 2005.
4. Flying the Hump to China, King S, AuthorHouse 2005.
5. ibid, Davidson.
6. ibid, Navigator's Log.

Serial Murder, Execution & LBJ's 'Peeping Tom'

Sometime this year or next, if he is still alive, William Heirens will again (for the 58th time) argue his annual plea for clemency before the Illinois parole board. Again, he is not likely to go free.

Heirens was a bright 17-year-old University of Chicago student when was arrested early in 1946 for petty burglary and suspicion of murder after taunting police in phone calls for failing to capture him. Using the made-up name of George Murman, he remained cocky when interrogated for several days, protesting innocence.

Then unexpectedly, he became talkative and helpful to detectives, admitting that he kidnapped, strangled, and dismembered six-year-old Suzanne Degnan. He also described strangling two young women. What caused the abrupt switch from quiet smart-ass to loquacious cooperation?

Even before the state's attorney announced the confession, the *Chicago Tribune*[1] was first to report it, noting that it was not the result of police brutality but after Heirens was injected with the "truth drug" sodium pentothal. At the ensuing trial I asked my chum on the Criminal Courts beat, assistant state's attorney William Tierney,* about the alleged injection.

He at first denied use of the drug, then conceded it was administered as part of a plea bargain to avoid the expense of a long trial. In return, Heirens would face three consecutive life terms in prison instead of execution. Another part of the deal was that he re-enact the murders. During the re-enactment, I tagged along with detectives on North Shore streets as Heirens showed how he lifted manhole covers and deposited Suzanne's body parts—an arm here, a leg there.

Did the trial judge, Harold Ward, know about the drug injection? I asked Tierney. "Sure," he replied, "and so did Heirens' public defender. It was all worked out in the judge's chambers. But if you quote me, I'll deny it." [2]

* Not his real name.

My city editor, Larry Mulay, decided not to mention this in the story because Judge Ward refused to confirm it. In fact, at parole hearings over the past half century, Heirens cited the sodium pentothal injection as a "contamination" of his conviction. He also claimed additional prosecutorial and police misconduct, incompetent defense counsel, false confession, and mistaken eyewitness identification.

Just as adamantly, authorities at the parole sessions repeatedly have denied injecting the drug and the prisoner's other allegations. Does this mean I am now obligated to appear on his behalf at the next clemency hearing? Bring on the subpoena.

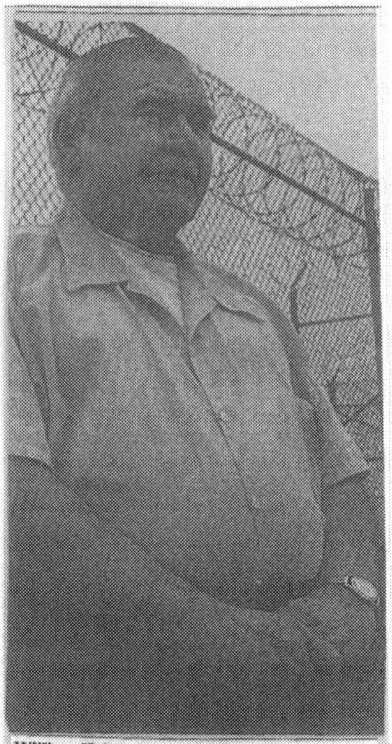

William Heirens outside Illinois prison in 2002. He repeatedly has sought release after serving more than half-century for three murders.
Photo by Peter Thompson for New York Times.

By late 2005, at age 77, Heirens was the longest serving inmate in the Illinois prison system. He was also the only serial killer in those years to have avoided the electric chair.

When There Is an Execution

In a typical execution, I would report from a viewing gallery at the Cook County jail, next to the courts building. Relatives of the convicted murderer, along with the family of the victim, prosecutors, police, and the defense attorney, also watched as the inmate was strapped to the specially wired chair, hooded, and electrocuted amid the jail's dimming lights.

Afterwards, warden Frank Sain, would lead us through his adjoining jail residence to a heaping buffet table. Most of the execution guests ate heartily, chatted amiably, and seemed to enjoy a macabre camaraderie. The scene still haunts me. Were these people a modern-day version of joyous mobs at a witch-burning or a lynching or a guillotining?

School of Hard Knocks & No Peeping Tom

News coverage of the Heirens and other stories about murder, including the "busman's holiday" scoop about the Denver man who dynamited an airliner,[3] typified a mind set that thrives on competing with oneself. I had done so in wartime by trying to achieve a better score of navigation of ETA (estimated time of arrival) and destination proximity than previous missions.

Returning to civilian work early in 1946 at the City News Bureau of Chicago, I pursued a comparable goal of self-competition. The stimulating day to day activity over a 12-year period blended CNB's 75-year tradition—described variously as "journalism's school of hard knocks" and "the reporter's boot camp"—with hands-on police and other beat coverage, feature writing, and hard-ass editing. That tradition produced alumni like novelist Kurt Vonnegut, multiple Pulitzer Prize winner Seymour Hersh, syndicated columnist Mike Royko, and playwright Charles MacArthur *(The Front Page.)*

In 1962, a distinguished journalist nearly fell victim to an erroneous police report. It began as a police radio call in CNB's newsroom: "Investigate a possible peeping tom on a fire escape" at a Northwest side apartment. Not an earth-shattering item for me, a copy boy, informing the city editor.

A responding police squad found that the man on the fire escape was for a breath of fresh air from a cigarette-smoking, rollicking party inside. There was no arrest, the police report noting that the man, *Chicago Daily News* reporter John Chancellor, was "not a peeping tom."

Hearing the same police radio call in the *Daily Times* newsroom was copy boy Jack Star, a former high school classmate of mine. He also spindled it.

Sixteen years later, the nonstory of 1946 resurfaced when Star, by now an assistant city editor (later to become a senior editor of *Look* magazine) fielded a telephone call from a man who said he was an FBI agent in Washington, D.C. Star confirmed the identity with a return call and was told, "This is a routine check on a John Chancellor, to head the USIA [United States Information Agency.] The boss, LBJ [President Lyndon B. Johnson], really wants him. Is it true he once was arrested as a peeping tom?"

Star related the true incident and soon afterwards, Chancellor took a leave of absence from news reporting at NBC to direct the USIA. When he returned to the television network a few years later, he was on a fast track as NBC-TV's evening news anchor.

One might say it was a lucky turn of events for Chancellor, from a falsely suspected Peeping Tom to a pinnacle of journalism. His successful career was not a result of chance. But in science and medicine, "chance" via serendipity plays a key role in what is often wrongly regarded as pure luck.

1. '40s Killer Seeks Release, Mill S., *Chicago Tribune,* Mar 4, 2002.

2. Personal communication.

3. See chapter on dynamiting of an airliner.

Serendipity—More Than 'Pure Luck'

How safety engineers click their tongues over that creature they call "accident prone." It seems he is forever crashing into automobiles, fouling up machinery, falling off ladders. But there is another kind of accident-prone individual who is dearly in demand.

He is the one who manages to make some valuable or pleasant discovery without deliberately looking for it. This ability is called serendipity, and it is broadening its smile of surprise throughout the fabric of medical progress.

Not long ago, for example, headlines announced that after a 25-year search, scientists at last had found a vaccine to prevent many cases of the common cold. But it was the discovery leader, ecologist Winston H. Price of the Johns Hopkins School of Hygiene and Public Health in Baltimore MD, looking for a cold preventive? He was not. Said Dr. Price: "We isolated the virus purely by luck. We weren't searching for it. It emerged through work on influenza."

Dr. Price is being modest of himself and his associates. While they had isolated a cold virus unintentionally, it took a high degree of perception, combined with thorough laboratory technique, to recognize the finding, verify it, and make the vaccine.

"Discoveries made by accident are never pure luck," said Dr. Robert Stormont, director of drug therapy and research at the American Medical Association,[1] when I interviewed him for a more detailed *JAMA* paper on serendipity. "They occur only because the individuals who make them are alert enough to fathom their usefulness. The key to how much future medical progress occurs may well be held by so-called odd-balls who depart from set-out tasks to look for unusual reactions from unusual substances."

After another Johns Hopkins researcher, allergist Leslie N. Gay, prescribed a new antihistamine, he noted this offhand comment from the patient: "By the way, doctor, this is the first time I haven't been dizzy or nauseated on the ride to your office." Throughout later tests of the drug, that casual remark figured prominently.

The result was dimenhydrinate (Dramamine), an effective motion sickness preventive. Some may call this a happy accident but it was no accident that an evaluative mind was able to grasp the significance of an apparently idle remark. On this deeper basis, medical history is filled with "happy accidents:"

The smallpox plague was conquered after Edward Jenner recalled the boast of a former milkmaid that she was immune because she had had cowpox—which then became the agent for mass immunity against smallpox.

A young physician, Rene Theophile Laennec, was looking only for relaxation one day in a Paris park where children were tapping "messages" to each other along opposite ends of a discarded plank He recognized in that game the principle that led to development of the stethoscope.

The alertness of another French physician, Auguste L. Loubatieres, also bore fruit. After treating typhoid patients with a sulfonamide, he noticed that the level of sugar in their blood dropped. So researchers tested a series of sulfonamide-like compounds. They wound up with tolbutamide, an orally given drug for diabetes mellitus.

Returning from a holiday to resume testing the potency of chicken cholera, Louis Pasteur accidentally inoculated some hens with a stale culture. His recognition of their resulting immunity through the action of "disarming" microbes became a foundation stone of preventive medicine. As Pasteur famously remarked, "Chance favors the prepared mind."[2]

These "happy accidents" have one point in common: Each was recognized, evaluated, and acted upon in the light of the discoverer's total intellectual experience. Pencillin offers perhaps the best illustration. As far back as the ninth century in Baghdad, the great Arab physician Rhazes was surprised to discover that putrefaction occurred to a greater degree in some parts of the city than in others. He could not have known that this was because concentrations of a mold called penicillium varied from place to place.

One thousand years later, in 1875, the physicist John Tyndall happened to notice differences in test tubes containing bacterial cultures. He wrote to the English Royal Society that "here was the slime of dormant or dead bacteria, the cause of their quiescence being the blanket of penicillium." But serendipity was not complete for Tyndall either; there was observation and recognition, but no pursuing action.

Tyndall's paper was forgotten—until a new generation in the person of Alexander Fleming made the same discovery, also "by accident," in 1928. It took the added perceptions of Howard W. Florey and Ernest B. Chain to show the tremendous medical import of Fleming's serendipity (all three shared the Nobel prize for medicine in 1945.)

And so our penicillin age is as much the fruit of 1,100 years' intellectual growth as it is the "luck" of multiple serendipity. As many a researcher will be first to admit, the fruit is still growing. Perspicacity is at an all-time premium. This is seen in more recent discoveries that have not yet been completely proved as true cases of serendipity. One concerns baboons, another involves rabbits and, still another, pink elephants in the sky:

A team of New York University-Bellevue scientists, engaged in rheumatic fever research, injected an enzyme called papaine (from the green papaya) into a rabbit. They were surprised to see the bunny's ears gradually wilt into the pose of a spaniel. While the experiment provided no help in the rheumatic fever study, chymopapaine's beneficial effect on cartilage helps other researchers in arthritis and other disorders.

Six baboons were stars of a serendipity incident in San Antonio, Texas. Dr. N. T. Werthessen of the Southwest Foundation for Research and Education began studying these apes, normally vegetarian, because of new clues that they were the only known animals that can develop atherosclerosis similar to the disease in humans. As he left his laboratory to take a trip, Dr. Werthessen blithely told the animal keeper, "Give 'em an ice cream and cake diet."

He said later, "It was just a figure of speech—I just meant to feed them well. But when I returned, I found that the baboons really were given ice cream and cake—and, to our surprise, they ate it. As every French pastry cook knows, ice cream will cover up the taste of most foods. So we began feeding them just about anything we please." This opened a new era of research: studying the effects of diet on heart disease.

Pink elephants, along with other hallucinations, began plaguing a teetotalling Swiss chemist named Hofmann as he was on his way home after doing some routine research with an ergot derivative called lysergic acid diethylamide. Recognizing that he may have been poisoned by the stuff, he later took a tiny measured dose and the effects were worse than before. Now this drug (LSD), which induces a schizophrenia-like condition, is proving valuable in mental health research.

While the promise of converting serendipity from a haphazard research method into a broadly tappable human resource remains a challenge, there always will be 'happy accident-prone" scientists—like the chemist who forgot to wash his hands before lunch. Having just worked with a strange substance, he wondered about the sugary taste of his roast beef sandwich.

He rushed back to his laboratory—to discover saccharine. It is the sweetest case of serendipity on record.

1. Serendipity—Big Word in Medical Progress, Golin M, *JAMA,* Dec 21, 1957.

2. Medicine's Happy Accidents, Golin M, *Yearbook Encyclopedia* 1959.

Near-Fatal Error, Sequester, Japanese Air Raid, and Seeking Amelia Earhart

While serendipity improved therapies that prevented deadly encounters, it could not prevent medical mishaps. Similarly, near-fatal error had been a constant peril in my wartime navigation missions. For example, on the last leg of a ferrying mission to Sardinia, from Algiers, navigation skills failed me. I goofed. This is what happened:[1]

Departure from Algiers was one hour behind, the island of Sardinia two hours ahead. The mid-day sky was overcast, affording no opportunity for sun or moon navigational aid. Wartime rules had silenced radio signal beacons.

Calculations at two10-minute intervals gave assurance of ground speed and course from the intensity and angle of Mediterranean Sea whitecaps below. Nothing unusual, except for a third drift meter reading that was rejected for indicating an impossibly high (70 mph) crosswind in seemingly smooth weather. No heavy turbulence.

Before rechecking for drift, I looked for signs of the sun piercing the overcast. No dice. By then it was time for a fourth drift reading. It confirmed the worst—a crosswind exceeding 60 miles an hour. The plane was perilously off course!

I rushed to the cockpit, shouted to the pilot, "Change heading to 37 degrees." Our unarmed B-26 "Marauder" bomber had been heading toward German-occupied Rome—to the city's concentration of anti-aircraft batteries and fighter plane squadrons.

The shouted alert came in the nick of time. After the landing in Sardinia,[2] analysis of weather patterns confirmed an unforecast squall line that had thrown the B-26 radically off course.At the same time, spotters on the island had caught sight of a Junkers JU-88, the celebrated German fighter-bomber-reconnaissance plane, far overhead at 26,000 feet.

"That guy's been following you," one spotter told me. The pilot had been tracking our B-26 during its windblown off-course route.

A Japanese Air Raid and Sequester in Yemen

A B-29 "Superfortress" bomber ferrying mission in1944 featured a Christmas night Japanese air raid that sent me leaping into a ditch during a refueling stop at a China airbase.[3] Confinement of crew had occurred three days earlier after one engine of the plane sprang an oil leak en route to a refueling point in Aden, Arabia.

The pilot, Lieut. James Conley, altered his heading to maneuver an emergency landing in Yemen at Salala. Troops armed with upraised scimitars surrounded the plane. An English-speaking officer explained that Yemen was a neutral nation in the war and therefore we must be sequestered.

To show "no hard feelings," he reached into baggy trousers and presented me with a large coin, along with an instant bit of Yemen history. "This is a Maria Teresa dollar, the world's purest silver coin," he said. "It has been our country's official currency for nearly a hundred years—since a ship off our coast sank with barrels of the coins. Yemeni salvage crews recovered most of them."

We spent the night in a large tent under guard. Our flight engineer was roused before dawn next morning to repair the oil leak, and we resumed the flight to Aden.

After Seven Years, Still Seeking Amelia Earhart

An October 23–30, 1944 mission to New Guinea from Oakland CA was considered especially hazardous. Because this was the first time that a squadron of heavily laden twin-engine planes, Curtiss-Wright C-46s, would be making the 2,150-mile first leg of the trip, the U.S. Navy had spaced four rescue vessels along the Pacific route. We landed at Hickam Field, Honolulu with no more than 60 gallons of fuel remaining.[4]

During the 1,000-mile leg from Canton Island to battle-scarred Tarawa, minor course diversions were ordered so that the crew could scan the waters and tiny islands en route for signs of Amelia Earhart or her plane.[5] She had vanished with navigator Fred Noonan during their round-the-world flight seven years earlier. Some aviation historians blamed poor navigation in the vicinity of Howland Island, on the equator about 200 miles east-southeast of Tarawa.

Earhart and Noonan had begun a long flight in the region with undetected compass error. They had another strike against them—relying on pre-war marine charts of the hundreds of Pacific islands, some of which years later were found to have been plotted as far as 20 miles from their true positions. Of course our C-46 crew found no clues to Earhart, Noonan, or their single-engine plane.

In trying to reach the destination of our ATC mission—Finchhaven, New Guinea—we experienced two potentially deadly confrontations with enemy troops. The first was a battle alert that lasted 20 minutes during a required low-altitude flight toward the airbase runway.

Briefing officers had told us that enemy forces lay in wait on both sides of the New Guinea combat corridor.[6] We were not attacked, however. Nor could we have returned fire since ferried aircraft typically are not armed or manned with gunners.

Relieved at the mission's conclusion, crew headed for the mess hall lines. Halfway to food at steam tables, three scruffy characters wearing low-visor caps tried to break into the line. Soldiers ahead of us let them in and when I yelled, "Hey, the line forms back here," a corporal nearby whispered, "It's OK. They're really hungry."

It turned out that the three scruff-necks were soldiers from an inactive Japanese encampment a mile away who each day would slip into the U.S. Army chow lines for sustenance—a routine that the GIs tolerated. It seemed that everybody knew this and nobody tried to capture the famished interlopers.

To critics of U. S. Air Transport Command crews for their relatively noncombatant status, we in the ATC could point to distinctive vulnerabilities. Fuel depletion during misguided or overly long missions was only one of the perils. There were also flights to and through combat zones in unarmed planes, targeting by enemy fighters and anti-aircraft batteries, and terrifying monsoon weather aloft.

Deadly encounters took on a different geographic dimension when the Air Transport Command diluted its force of ferrying navigators—particularly those certified in meteorology—to a more urgent need: airlifting vital aviation fuel and troops to repel Japanese invaders in China.

Too many of the transport planes between India/Burma and China airbases were being lost, largely because of safety lapses blamed on poor briefings and weather forecasts. And so now a new navigational challenge began—from long-distance ferrying to weather analysis and route planning for hazardous flights across the Himalayan "Hump,"[6] (as described in the "danger and diversion" chapter.)

Slipping into a White House Reception—for an Exclusive

The contrasting interval between a 1944 New Guinea war zone and a peaceful White House scene 30 years later could not have been more stark. Here in 1974, nobody was gunning for anyone. There were no deadly encounters (although lobbyists schmoozed in deadly earnest), no areas of conflict. This was the fun time of a Presidential party, and of a reporter seeking a news scoop.

Overhead floodlights of the White House north portico glowed on colorful gowns, shiny tuxedo sashes, and muted conversation. The line of guests snaked to and through the open gate of the wrought iron fence, along the path of low shrubbery, and up the steps toward the ballroom. Engraved invitations in the hands of some were scanned cursorily by Secret Service agents. They smilingly waved in other guests whose faces permitted entry. Music from a string ensemble wafted into the chill of December 1974.

Inside was an expanded scene of pomp and color: Bejeweled women in formal gowns, escorted by men in business or formal wear, Army and Air Force generals and Navy admirals with tiers of battle ribbons, a few foreign diplomats whose companions whisked by in mauve or pink saris.

Maneuvering across the ballroom floor between clusters of guests, young men clad in tuxedos held trays of champagne flutes, hors d'oeuvres, and small sandwiches. Two crystal chandeliers sparkled high above. Having skipped both breakfast and lunch that day, I reached for two of the tiny sandwiches and washed down both with champagne. The musicians, I noticed, were alternating Broadway show tunes and Mozart selections.

Near them, bracketed by two U. S. Marines in dress blues, stood the stars of the reception, President Gerald R Ford and his vice presidential designate, Nelson A. Rockefeller. They were greeting guests who were winding back through an adjoining ballroom. The same waiter approached with more food and drink. This time I slipped one of the sandwiches into my jacket pocket and consumed another with more champagne.

From the drift of conversation, it soon became apparent that many of the guests were Senate and House leaders, and others were from large corporations and labor groups. One voice over a bowtie asked, "Has U. S. Steel seen the subcommittee's latest draft?" Lobbyists.

Here was an opportunity to end my lack of companionship. "Excuse me," I addressed the group, "but I couldn't help overhearing. For years I've been trying to reach a college friend, William Ahlfeld. Last I heard, he was PR director at U. S. Steel."

"Sure, I know Bill," another bowtie said, reaching into a pocket for a business card. "He's still with us. Call me next week and I'll put you in touch."

What was I doing in this scene of glamour and opulence? I asked myself. I knew the answer perfectly well. Yesterday I had premeditated crashing the reception after learning that a pool of only three reporters—from the *New York Times, Washington Post,* and Associated Press—would be allowed entry by the White House press office. Why only the "big" media?

Which was why I'd put aside my tweed sports jacket this morning and worn the navy blue suit. There was little likelihood that the eagle-eyed press secretary, Ron Nesson, positioned with the Secret Service men on the portico, would recognize me. I had been only an occasional attendee at White House press briefings. Certainly I had a right to be here, defying the discriminatory press pool rule. This was my beat.

There was no doubt, though, that uninvited presence was risking my White House credentials. Three months earlier, those credentials had opened entry to the Oval Office after a press assistant announced to correspondents in the downstairs briefing room, "Photo opportunity!"

Cameras in hand, we trotted along a corridor to find President Ford seated with advisors and an Israeli delegation. I snapped pictures of him, Henry Kissinger, and prime minister Itzhak Rabin. Standing alert against a wall was a Rabin bodyguard, whose Uzi automatic pistol bulged noticeably from the breast pocket of his jacket.

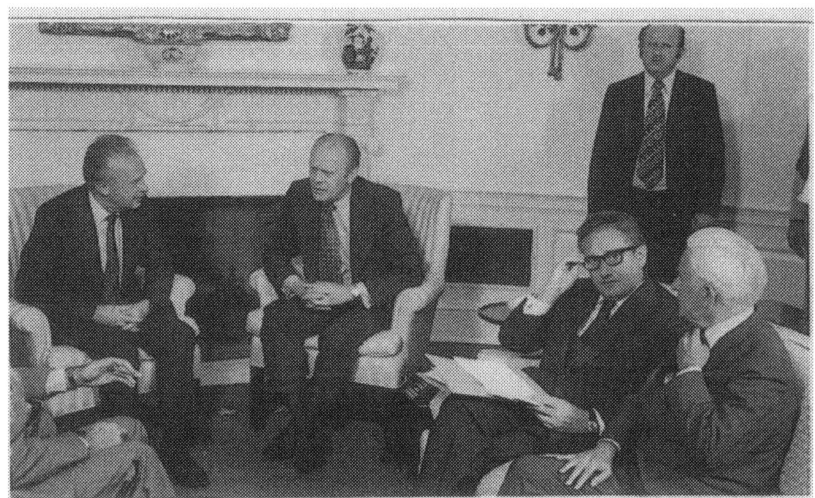

Oval Office conference with Israeli delegation Sept. 11, 1974. Bracketing president Gerald Ford are Israel prime minister Itzhak Rabin and secretary of state Henry Kissinger. Man at far right is unidentified. Standing is Mossad bodyguard, his jacket breast pocket bulging with Uzi pistol. *Photo by White House correspondent Milton Golin, copyright 1974.*

(Holding my camera case was a guest correspondent from Chicago, former AMA colleague Carol Brierly of *American Medical News.* A year later, having both been widowed, we were married. We still are.

At the Presidential reception, my friend the tuxedoed sandwich man approached again. I wasn't fooling him. When I reached for two, he advised under his breath, "Take another. They're small." More for the side pocket. Now another challenge: the President's greeting line. Within ten seconds, I spotted a gap and slipped into it.

Directly in front, chatting with a jovial couple, was Caspar Weinberger, the Secretary of Health, Education and Welfare. Behind me, unaccompanied and looking as if he might welcome a bit of conversation, was Supreme Court Chief Justice Warren Burger. A large bandage on part of his left hand stuck out like, well, a sore thumb. That's exactly what it was, a sore thumb.

"Ouch," I said. "That must hurt."

"Not much now. But there was pain over the weekend."

Mr. Justice Burger, I remembered, had been a member of the Mayo Clinic board of trustees, the country's second largest doctor-run group practice, after Kaiser. So here might be an item for my publication, *Medical Group News.*

The interview began. But here was no place for conventional note taking, not even with my special method[1] contributed to the book *A Treasury of Tips for Writers.* This had to be questions and answers committed to memory.

Q—What happened?
A—Ran my bike into a parked car in front of my home.
Q—You hit the pavement?
A—Oh yes. My wife saw it from the front doorway.
Q—Did she call 911?

A—Started to but changed her mind. Rushed over as neighbors were helping me up. One of them wheeled the bike next to my driveway as she pulled out the car to drive me to the hospital [in suburban Virginia.]

Q—Any broken bones?
A—The ER doctors don't think so. But they put in a stiff piece to prevent damage.
Q—Just like back at Mayo, right?
A—Have we met before?
Q—No, but the Clinic has been receiving *Medical Group News.* .I'm Milt Golin, the editor.
A—Oh, yes
Q—Are you recuperating at home?
A—No need to. This morning, though, Lewis wisecracked that this bandage should stop me from hitchhiking to work. [Lewis was Justice Lewis Powell Jr., also an ex-Mayo Clinic trustee.]

By now, the friendly chatter behind us had stopped while others in the receiving line seemed to be hanging onto Mr. Chief Justice Burger's every word. Also, Secretary Weinberger had reached the Marine guard and identified himself.

Most in the receiving line saw the guard whisper Weinberger's name into President Ford's ear. Protocol. For Weinberger, of course, this was not necessary.

"Good to see you, Cap," the president said. "Historic event, wouldn't you say?" I was next. The guard whispered to Ford, "Milton Golin, publisher of Medical Group News."

"Welcome," the president boomed. "Enjoy the evening." His handshake was not the dead fish of Richard Nixon at past Christmas parties for White House correspondents, but a firm and strong grip like a football player's. Ford had in fact been a college halfback.

Now, my identity for the next Marine guard, alongside Mr. Rockefeller. The greeting was "Thanks for being here.This is quite an occasion." The string ensemble was ending a Mozart sonata and launching into a tune from *South Pacific.* Waiters with champagne and food again looked inviting to me.

After downing the drink, finishing off one tiny ham and cheese and pocketing another, I wondered how I could have figured there were only two glass chandeliers overhead. There had to be at least six. The unsober view told me it was time to leave. Musicians were moving into a Mozart rondo.

A few guests were saying their goodbyes, even as more were arriving. Ron Nesson was still on the portico eagle-eyed, along with his two Secret Service buddies. We made eye contact and again he made no sign of recognition.

Only a bit unsteadily, I headed for the north gate exit. Outside, a couple of dozen onlookers craned their necks, apparently seeking celebrity faces. A middle-aged, well-dressed woman thrust one arm through the iron fence bars as I approached and asked, "Please?"

In her hand were a ballpoint pen and a copy of *Playbill.* I guessed that she had stepped out of the National Theater two blocks away during an intermission and decided to check out the limousines snailing toward 1600 Pennsylvania Avenue.

"Sure," I said and, with a flourish, wrote "David O. Lilienthal," purposefully faking the middle initial. I did the same for a young man in a jacket with leather elbow patches when he proffered a small spiral notebook.

During the drive home to Bethesda, I polished off the hoarded sandwiches. Next morning at the office, I described the exhilarating White House episode to editorial aide Dorothy ("Duffy") Miller. Her first question was, "How did you come up with the David Lilienthal identity?"

"I don't know. The name just popped up in my head."

"So any day now, at an autograph convention," said Duffy, "somebody's going to hold up that name and brag about a rare signature from the head of the Atomic Energy Commission."

It was page layout deadline for *Medical Group News.* We lifted a four-inch item from the front page, moved it into space inside, and substituted a summary of the brief Chief Justice Burger interview. The word *Exclusive,* in not too flashy 10 point italics, was placed above the headline:

Chief Justice Burger,
Former Mayo Trustee,
Hurt in Bike Mishap

No earth-shaking exclusive, to be sure. But after scanning the news columns of both big Washington newspapers for the past week, as well as the society pages (where we all knew the "real" news often originated) I was confident we alone had the story. It was a scoop.

1. *A Treasury of Tips for Writers*, Weisbrod M, ed. Writer's Digest Books 1965.

References

Title Pages

1. Behind the Front Page, Dornfeld AA,
   Academy Chicago Press 1983.

Louisiana Hurricane

1. Saga of the Disaster Doctors,
   Golin M *JAMA* Aug 10,1957

Deadly Thought

1. How Deadly the Thought, Golin M, *JAMA,* Sep 12, 1959.

2. Is Neurosis Catching?, Golin M., *Charm,* April 1959.

Religion & Medicine

1. Near Life, Near Death, Near God, Golin M, *JAMA,* Apr 13, 1957 *Reader's Digest,* Sep 1957.

2. ibid.

3. Personal communication.

4. Bringing Doctors to Main Street, *Reader's Digest,* Jan 1957.

5. See Footnote 1.

6. AMA Newsletter, Nov 20, 1957.

Wartime Mutiny

1. Letters to and from U.S. Air Force historian P. Hallion, archivist Archie Difante. and medical research Commander Col. Carol S. Sikes.

2. Air Navigation Log of M. Golin. World map ATC missions of M. Golin.

3. ibid. navigation log.

4. ibid. navigation log.

5. ibid.

6. See footnote 1.

7. ibid.

8. A Mutiny of One, Kurson R, Chicago *Magazine,* June 2002.

Teddy Roosevelt's Savior

1. Chicago's Forgotten Hero, Golin M, *Coronet Magazine* March 1951.

Not Baby Sitters

1. Don't Call Them Baby Sitters, Golin M, *Saturday Evening Post,* Jun 20, 1959.

Colorado Bombing

1. Dynamiter Denies Story, Nakulla A, *Rocky Mountain News,* Nov 18, 1955.

2. Guilt Denied in Plane Bombing, *New York Times,* Nov 19, 1955.

3. Plane Bomber Gets Delay, AP *Chicago Tribune,* Nov 18, 1955.

4. 4. Behind the Front Page, Dornfeld AA, Academy Chicago Publishers, 1983

5. ibid. *Rocky Mountain News.*

6. Turner and Golin Take Bus Driver's Holiday, RTNDA Newsletter, Jan 56 Illinois News Broadcasters Assn Newsletter, Jan 1956.

Autistic Kids

1. Autism: The Internet As Haven, Educator, Social Catalyst, & Therapeutic Key, Golin M, Computers & *Medicine,* Aug 1997.

Mars Rescue

1. The Moon Is Old Hat, Golin M., *JAMA,* Jan 31, 1959.

2. Health in the Heavens, *JAMA* "Medicine at Work," Jun 15, 1957.

Danger and Diversion

1. Air Navigator's Log Book

2. Self-published diary of W. Davidson 1978.

3. ibid., Hump Pilots Assn. 2002 newsletter.

4. Flying the Hump to China, King S, AuthorHouse 2005.

5. ibid. Davidson.

6. .ibid. navigator's log.

Serial Murder…

1. '40s Serial Killer Seeks Release, Mills S, *Chicago Tribune,* Mar 4, 2002.

2. Personal communication.

3. See chapter 5.

4. Behind the Front Page, Dornfeld AA, Academy Chicago Publishers 1983.

5. Personal communication.

Serendipity

1. Serendipity—Big Word in Medical Progress, Golin M, *JAMA,* Dec 21, 1957.

2. Medicine's Happy Accidents, Golin M, Yearbook Encyclopedia 1959.

Near-Fatal Error

1. Air Navigation Log of Lt. M. Golin

2. ibid. log and map.

3. ibid.

4. ibid. navigator's log

5. Flight to Everywhere: A Navigator's Life, Farmer M, Coralreef Group 1998.

6. ibid.

Presidenial Reception

1x. See illustration

1. A Treasury of Tips for Writers, Weisbrod M, ed, Writer's Digest Books 1965.

Author Biography

Who's Who in Midwest, Marquis, 1998–99
Who's Who in Healthcare, Hanover Publicxations
Reader's Guide to Periodicals Lit. 1966–7-
Chicago City News Bureau archives
Journal AMA library and archives
U.S. Army Air Forces discharge.
U.S. Secret Service (White House correspondent accreditation).

Among 29 JAMA Papers by Assistant Editor Milton Golin

How Little Towns Get Good Doctors*	Sep 29, 1956
The Automobile: A Challenge to Medicine	Oct 27, 1956
Doctors Who Talk About War (civil defense)	Nov 14, 1956
Music As a Medical Tool*	Dec 29, 1956
Pursuing the Killers (poison control centers)*	Jan 12, 1957
Is There a Doctor in the Plant? (occupational medicine)*	Mar 30, 1957
Near Life, Near Death, Near God (religion and medicine)*	Apr 13, 1957
How Authentic Is Medicine on Television?*	May 4, 1957
Health in the Heavens (aerospace medicine)*	Jun 15, 1957
Medicine's Biggest Battle: Taming Time (aging)	Jul. 27, 1957
Saga of the Disaster Doctors (hurricane)*	Aug 10, 1957
Bootstraps for Our Forgotten Millions (disability rehab)	Nov. 2, 1957
Serendipity—Big Word in Medical Progress*	Dec 21, 1957
Robber of Five Million Brains (alcoholism)*	Jul. 19, 1958
The Troubled Employee*	Nov. 8, 1958
The Moon is 'Old Hat' (interview with space doctor)*	Jan. 31, 1958
Snow Emergency!	Feb. 21, 1958
How One Physician Warned a Nation (plastic bags hazard)*	Apr 25, 1958

** Reprints or digests in other national periodicals. Papers average 4,500 words.*

About the Author

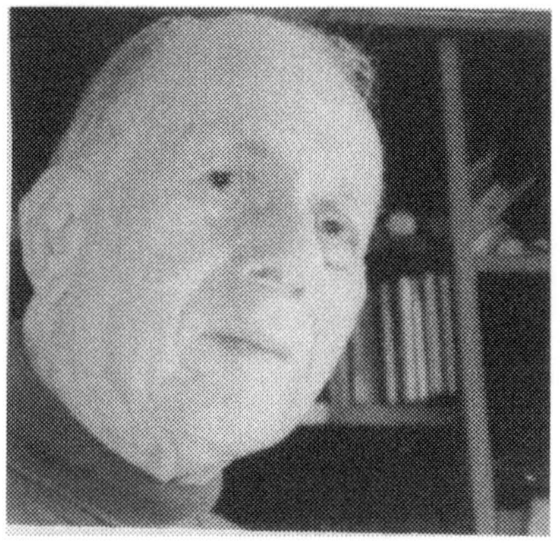

After World War II service as a U.S. Air Force navigator, Milton Golin resumed working as a Chicago news reporter. Later he became the first nonphysician assistant editor of *The Journal of the American Medical Association.* This led to assignments in Washington, DC as an accredited White House correspondent. Golin's articles have appeared in over 200 newspapers and national magazines. He earned campaign ribbons with three bronze battle stars for action in six theaters of war. He and his wife Carol Brierly Golin, also a journalist, live near downtown Chicago.

Epilogue

Hurricane Katrina on August 27, 2005, whose deaths and destruction make it the worst storm in American history, might be just a recent example of natural crises that lie ahead.

Long-range weather forecasters expect a sharply rising number of hurricanes in the next decade. Add these to more predicted forest fires and earthquakes, and the challenge is clear to two groups of professionals: doctors and news reporters.

Along with civil defense and rescue teams, they have been in the forefront of disaster scenes [see chapter 1]. Why? Because practicing physicians and working journalists traditionally experience comparable high drama in deadly encounters.

The doctor ministers to the critical-care patient at a hospital bedside, during a natural disaster, in an epidemic, on a battlefield, around a severe accident. At the same time and place, the skilled reporter serves readers and viewers by accurately and meaningfully portraying the medical efforts.

Little wonder, then, that the diligent journalist whose aim is to seek a fresh approach to a news story is on a par with the innovative physician's search for correct diagnoses and treatments. This book confirms the mutual goals.

Continuing to do so illustrates that doctors at work coincide with investigative reporters at work—in time for their next emergency call.

Acknowledgements

So many people in varying roles figured in the genesis and outcome of this book that it is hard knowing where laudable words should begin. At the outset, two women friends—Oklahoma City history buff and educator Anne Hathcote and Sarasota, FL mathematics aficionado Ila Stone—were the first to persist with "Write it down!" after hearing about what became the chapter on my wartime armed mutiny.

Echoing their urgings was John J. Nance of Tacoma, WA, an airline pilot and aeronautics consultant for ABC-TV News. He recalled during a 2001 St. Paul MN safety conference that his father, like me, had been a B-25 aviator in World War II.

Among physicians who have shared their insight and experience in research, practice, and medical education have been: retired chest physician Dr. Ray Hillson, pilot of a still-operating B-25 bomber in Aurora, IL; Dr. Monroe Richman of Kaloa, HI, medical essayist extraordinaire; Chicago interventional cardiologist Dr. James Flaherty; Dr. Raja Khuri, a retired professor at Northwestern University's medical school, medical administrator Dr. Fred Featherstone and acclaimed cardiothoracic surgeon Dr. Patrick .M. McCarthy.

Also, special thanks for advice from fellow members of the American Society of Journalists and Authors including Murray Teigh Bloom, Lynn Lamberg, Charles Remsberg, and Barbara Goodheart; former *Look* magazine senior editor and longtime mentor-by-example Jack Star; and retired McGraw-Hill executive Marvin Rowlands and Miller. Plaudits, too, for pro-duction help from Mike Altman of iUniverse and from Laura Hill for picture processing.

This book received a vital jump-start from *Chicago* editor Richard Babcock and best-selling author *(Shadow Divers)* Robert Kurson. Their June, 2002 magazine story of my wartime mutiny set the stage for other chapters.

Compiling the 450-plus entries for the index draws plaudits for son James Golin. A devotee of trivia, he notes that among names listed are those of five American presidents, two justices of the U. S. Supreme Court, and more than a half-dozen world class scientists—not to mention Amelia Earhart, Henry Kissinger, Jimmy Doolittle, Bill Gates, Itzhak Rabin, and Douglas MacArthur.

Nor was Jim the only close relative to contribute. Stepdaughter Amy Brierly not only introduced the B-25 pilot/physician Ray Hillson but also showed her publicist skills and instilled in me her expertise in helping to highlight the public service thrusts of the daring doctors. The supreme family input came from wife Carol Brierly Golin, a Phi Beta Kappa investigative journalist in her own right. Carol's keen eye for get-go substance versus triviality in story telling has been invaluable—particularly amid her unflagging counsel, inspiration, and support during difficult moments of typescripting *Daring Docs.** With allies like these, what author could ask for more?

* Carol has had her own daring moments. At age four, along with other dance-school pupils, she performed with fan dancer Sally Rand at Chicago's Century of Progress world's fair. But that's another true story for telling.

Index

978-0-595-38194-4
0-595-38194-4

www.ingramcontent.com/pod-product-compliance
Ingram Content Group UK Ltd.
Pitfield, Milton Keynes, MK11 3LW, UK
UKHW041936190726
13854UKWH00004B/1623